The
MACULAR
DEGENERATION
Source Book

A GUIDE for PATIENTS and FAMILIES

Bert Glaser, M.D.
Lester A. Picker, Ed.D.

Addicus Books
Omaha, Nebraska

An Addicus Nonfiction Book

ISBN 1-886039-53-4
Cover design by George Foster
Illustrations by Mark Gibson and Jack Kusler

This book is not intended to be a substitute for a physician, nor do the authors intend to give advice contrary to that of an attending physician.

Library of Congress Cataloging-in-Publication Data
Glaser, Bert, 1949-
  The macular degeneration source book : a guide for patients and
families / Bert Glaser, Lester A. Picker.
      p. cm.
Includes bibliographical references and index.
   ISBN 1-886039-53-4
   1. Retinal degeneration—Popular works. I. Picker, Lester A., 1947-
II. Title.
   RE661.D3 G56 2001
   617.7'35—dc21
                                        2001003462

Addicus Books, Inc.
P.O. Box 45327
Omaha, Nebraska 68145
Web site: http://www.AddicusBooks.com

Printed in the United States of America
10 9 8 7 6 5 4 3 2 1

To my wife Ronnie, who is my anchor,
and my sons Eric and Harris, who are my inspiration.

Bert Glaser, M.D.

To my wife Leslie, who brings love and joy to my life; to our
collective children—Jennifer, Matthew, Melissa, Aaron,
Christie, and Neil—who have taught me much about life;
and to our grandchildren—Matthew, Tonya,
Aidan, Ananda, William, and Terran—who have blessed us with
the unadulterated bliss of being grandparents.

Lester A. Picker, Ed.D.

Contents

Acknowledgments

As a physician, I am acutely aware of the natural desire of patients to understand their condition. I am also very aware of the great difficulty patients encounter when they attempt to get accurate and understandable information. As a result, I have wanted to produce clearly written explanations of medical conditions for my patients. Although I have considerable expertise in the diagnosis and management of retinal disorders and have written hundreds of articles in professional journals, as well as numerous chapters in medical textbooks, I am not an expert in writing for a non-medical audience. Therefore, I needed a partner who could understand complex medical information and help me translate it into a format that would be easily understood by non-medical readers. A unique set of qualities would be required. I have been blessed to find this partner—Lester Picker. In addition to his great skills as a communicator, Les shares my enthusiasm for medical science and my compassion for people suffering from medical conditions.

An understandable explanation of complex systems often hinges on well-designed illustrations. Jack Kusler and Mark Gibson, who illustrated this book, have the ability to grasp complex concepts and translate them into illuminating illustrations. We thank them.

Much of what I have been able to accomplish in my career has been aided by the lessons learned from my late teacher and partner, Dr. Ronald G. Michels. Dr. Michels embodied the best of clinical skill, intellectual honesty, curiosity, and integrity. He remains my guiding light.

I also thank Dr. Jack Skeen for his friendship and his willingness to always shine a light into the darkness so that I may better see the truth.

Bert Glaser, M.D.

When Dr. Bert Glaser and I first discussed collaborating on this book, he said something that will stay with me forever. "I live in the fovea," he remarked, referring to the part of the retina, tinier than the period at the end of this sentence, where macular degeneration does its damage.

At the time I thought the comment a bit odd, but I soon came to appreciate the passion for his work that drives Bert Glaser. I have never met a physician so dedicated to his craft and science, nor such an enthusiastic teacher. He typically spends twelve to sixteen hours a day performing delicate laser surgery on the retina through a microscope, and is deeply concerned for his patients. He is a pioneering researcher, using state-of-the-art techniques, yet he is also an old-fashioned doctor, seeing his patients as whole human beings. As a result, this book was a joy to write from beginning to end. And, one thing I learned for sure. Should I ever need a retinal surgeon, I will let no one else but Bert near my eyes.

Acknowledgments

I quickly came to appreciate the commitment that publisher Rod Colvin of Addicus Books brings to his work. Through several drafts of the manuscript, Rod focused on how to bring the most value to our readers.

Most of all, I thank God for bringing my wife, Leslie, into my life. Her support, encouragement, and loving smile were instrumental in bringing this work to life.

Lester A. Picker, Ed.D.

Introduction

A new case of macular degeneration is diagnosed every three minutes in the United States, according to the Macular Degeneration Foundation. As a physician, medical researcher and surgeon specializing in diseases of the retina, I help people every day who are suffering from the effects of macular degeneration. Both patients and their families want an easy-to-understand guide that explains its causes, how to prevent or slow its progress, and the most effective treatments now available.

For the first time in decades, there is new hope for patients with macular degeneration. Scientists from diverse fields have made pioneering advances in our understanding of this debilitating disease. Each finding solves one mystery about macular degeneration and leads to new lines of promising research. For example, we now have new ways to examine the tiny vessels that supply the retina with nutrient-rich blood. In fact, I have been a pioneer in the use of special dyes that enable retinal surgeons to see and treat the leaking blood vessels that cause macular degeneration. These techniques have dramatically improved our ability to surgically stem the effects of macular degeneration.

Entirely new categories of drugs show promise for slowing the damaging effects of macular degeneration. There is also increasing attention being given today to new methods that may soon allow us to transplant healthy retinas to those patients whose retinas have been damaged by macular degeneration. There is even a great deal of research being conducted on how nutrition might prevent a person from ever getting the disease.

In this book I attempt to separate fact from fiction, hype from true hope. Unfortunately, at present, there is no cure for macular degeneration. But there are things one can do to slow its development and to adjust better to the challenges it presents.

Finally, medical science changes our understanding of diseases very quickly. As specialists in diseases of the retina, my staff and I stay abreast of the latest developments in the field. To provide my patients and readers of my book with the latest information, I have created a Web site that is constantly updated (www.glasermurphyretina.com). So, please accept my invitation to research information on macular degeneration, to just browse, to join one of the discussion groups, to share your experiences, or to send me an E-mail.

It is my sincerest hope that you and your family will benefit from this book.

1

Macular Degeneration: An Overview

Some 15 million Americans suffer from the visual impairments of macular degeneration, and more than 200,000 new cases are recorded every year. It is the most common cause of vision loss in Americans over age 50. Although a person has only a 2 percent chance of getting macular degeneration while in his or her fifties, that risk increases to nearly 30 percent after age 75, according to the National Eye Institute. With the aging of baby boomers, the number of individuals diagnosed with macular degeneration is expected to rise significantly.

What Is Macular Degeneration?

Macular degeneration is an abnormality in the blood supply to a portion of the retina known as the macula. As a result, one's central vision deteriorates. There are two basic types of macular degeneration: dry and wet. In *dry macular degeneration*, which affects about 90 percent of patients, the blood supply to the retina is diminished. In *wet macular degeneration*, which affects the other 10 percent of those diagnosed, the blood supply is excessive.

The Normal Eye

To better understand how macular degeneration develops, it is important to understand the basic anatomy of the back portion of the eye.

The *retina* is an extremely thin and delicate sheet of tissue, with the consistency of wet tissue paper. It sits on the back, inner surface of the eye and is responsible for detecting the image that is focused on it by the *lens*. Like film in a camera, the retina must be absolutely flat in order to provide clear, undistorted vision. Any unevenness or irregularity of the retina will result in distortion and/or blurring of vision.

The *macula* is the small, central area of the retina that is responsible for reading and other visual tasks requiring the detection of fine detail, such as recognizing faces at a distance and

Cross Section of Eyeball

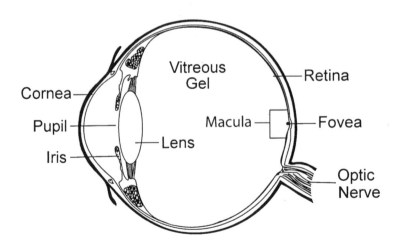

Normal Retina

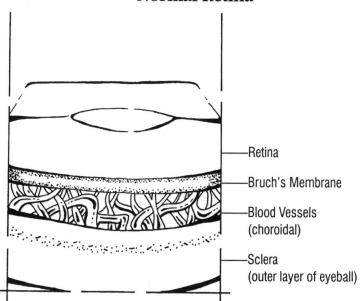

In the normal eye, the blood passes through the Bruch's membrane, supplying nourishment to the retina.

reading street signs. If the retina as a whole were a target, the macula would be the bull's-eye. Within the macula sits the most sensitive portion, the *fovea.* The fovea is so tiny, it would easily fit within the period at the end of this sentence.

In the healthy eye, the retina lies over a flat carpet of blood vessels that provides it with nourishment. Between the retina and those blood vessels is a thin, compact layer of fibers called *Bruch's membrane,* which provides support and elasticity to help prevent damage to the delicate retinal tissue. Nutrients traveling from the blood vessels to the retina must pass through Bruch's membrane. In the normal eye, Bruch's membrane does not impede this crucial flow of nutrients.

The Aging Eye

The retina is continually working. During our waking hours it processes light images constantly, consuming lots of energy and nutrients, processing them, and generating waste products. Even as we sleep, the retina is working, repairing damage to its cells and storing energy. Much of the nutrients the retina requires come from the blood vessels underlying Bruch's membrane. They pass through the membrane to the retina. Conversely, waste products generated by the retina pass through Bruch's membrane on the way back to the blood vessels to be transported away.

As we age, some of these waste products accumulate within the fibers of Bruch's membrane. This debris can form into small yellow mounds called *drusen.* Although it's believed that all people accumulate some debris within Bruch's membrane during their lifetime, not all people will develop drusen that are visible to a physician during eye examinations. The continued accumulation of debris within the layers of Bruch's membrane thickens it, moving the retina further away from its blood supply and interfering with the transfer of nutrients. Bruch's membrane tends to get gummed up over time. This thickening and interference from drusen can contribute to macular degeneration.

Dry Macular Degeneration

When reduced blood flow to the retina results in a lack of nourishment to the tissue, many of the retinal cells gradually waste away. This process, which occurs most commonly in the macular (central) area of the retina, results in dry macular degeneration.

Dry Macular Degeneration

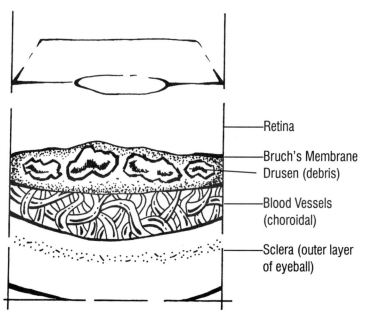

—Retina

—Bruch's Membrane
— Drusen (debris)

—Blood Vessels
(choroidal)

—Sclera (outer layer
of eyeball)

Dry macular degeneration occurs when debris, or drusen, collects within the fibers of the Bruch's membrane, impeding the blood flow to the retina.

This leads to blurred vision but usually does not cause rapid, severe visual loss.

The goal in treating dry macular degeneration is to prevent or reduce the formation of debris within Bruch's membrane and thereby maintain or improve the flow of nutrients to the retina from its underlying blood vessels.

Wet Macular Degeneration

Wet macular degeneration is a result of the eye growing new blood vessels to improve the blood flow to the retinal tissue. But, these new blood vessels may eventually leak blood or fluids under the retina. This leakage causes a blister to develop under the retina, usually in the macula. This part of the retina then becomes elevated and uneven. Images sent to the retina fall on the uneven surface, resulting in distorted and blurred vision. These disturbances in vision can occur very rapidly.

One of the great medical mysteries of wet macular degeneration has been finding out what causes these blood vessels to grow so rapidly toward the retina. Researchers now suspect that the retina, starved for nutrients, most likely sends out biochemical signals that call for new blood vessels. These new blood vessels also secrete *enzymes* that dissolve the tissue in their path, allowing them to grow into Bruch's membrane.

Medical studies have shown that as we age blood vessels grow into Bruch's membrane all the time; it is only a matter of degree as to whether a patient gets too few blood vessels, resulting in dry macular degeneration, or too many, resulting in wet.

Types of Wet Macular Degeneration

As new blood vessels migrate toward the retina, they cause varying disease features and symptoms. Knowing which type of wet macular degeneration you have can help you understand why certain treatments are suggested.

Classic Blood Vessel Formation

The first major type of wet macular degeneration is known as *classic*. In this form of the disease, excess blood vessels rapidly leak blood or fluids into the eye tissue under the retina; these tissues are essential to central vision. Classic macular degeneration

Wet Macular Degeneration

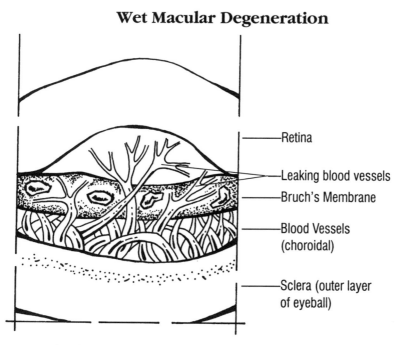

Retina

Leaking blood vessels

Bruch's Membrane

Blood Vessels (choroidal)

Sclera (outer layer of eyeball)

Wet macular degeneration is the result of blood vessels leaking blood or fluid under the retina, causing a blister to develop, usually under the macula.

is part of the leaking pattern in approximately 30 to 40 percent of all cases diagnosed. Pure classic is seen in only 1 percent of all cases. If left untreated, vision can deteriorate rapidly.

Occult Blood Vessel Formation

A slower leakage is known as *occult* macular degeneration. Approximately 96 percent of all cases of macular degeneration are predominantly occult or a mix of occult and classic. With occult, only a small amount of fluid is involved, so the retina is not as elevated and is not sending out as strong biochemical signals for more blood vessels. Since the macula is the area most typically involved, the patient experiences blurring and distortions in central vision.

Left untreated, occult macular degeneration causes visual loss more slowly than does the classic form, often taking weeks to months before it results in decreased vision. Occult will occasionally stop leaking by itself, while classic almost never stops leaking on its own. In addition, it is possible for occult to progress to classic.

Other Types of Macular Degeneration

Other types of macular degeneration are recognized by retinal specialists, but together they represent only a small fraction of total cases. These other forms may involve thinning of the retina, hemorrhages within the retina, scarring of the retina, and tears in or detachment of the *retinal pigment epithelium* (*RPE*), a single layer of cells between the retina and underlying blood vessels.

In one of these forms of macular degeneration, *polypoidal CNV*, little swellings occur within the newly grown blood vessels. These swellings weaken the walls of the blood vessels. The vessels can then burst and cause massive bleeding. This condition tends to occur more commonly in people of African-American and Middle Eastern heritage, with some estimates showing that perhaps 7 or 8 percent of these populations will have this form. In general, African-Americans and Middle Eastern people have a much lower rate of macular degeneration than Caucasians. Due to the risk of hemorrhaging from these swellings in the blood vessels, people in these two populations should be especially careful about monitoring their retinas and to have eye exams more frequently if they are ever diagnosed with macular degeneration.

Possible Side Effect of Eye Hemorrhaging

In a small percentage of macular degeneration cases, hemorrhages can bleed into the *vitreous*, a clear jelly-like substance that fills the back portion of the eye. This type of bleeding is called a vitreous hemorrhage. Although it is not a form of macular degeneration, a vitreous hemorrhage is an infrequent side effect of the bleeding that may accompany macular degeneration. It is critically important to understand that such a hemorrhage can cause sudden loss of both central vision and peripheral vision.

On the positive side, if a vitreous hemorrhage is detected early—within a few weeks—it can be remedied. The blood-stained vitreous can be removed, and in many cases, peripheral vision restored. The key is to get treatment as quickly as possible. If a few months pass without treatment, the blood in the vitreous can produce scarring, which results in permanent loss of vision.

2

Symptoms of Macular Degeneration

Macular degeneration presents a unique set of symptoms. Unfortunately, patients often wait too long before seeking treatment for this debilitating disease. It is critically important that people detect the early warning signs of macular degeneration and then seek treatment *immediately*. The sooner a person is treated for symptoms, the better the chances of arresting further deterioration or possibly even improving vision.

Initial Symptoms

Dry Macular Degeneration

Here, symptoms may include decreased vision, blurred vision, or darkened vision. Dry macular degeneration usually starts with blurring in the central field of vision and commonly progresses over a period of months or years. However, when people with dry macular degeneration experience distortion in their central field of vision, it often signals conversion to wet macular degeneration. In fact, any rapid change in symptoms over a period of days to weeks in people with dry macular degeneration usually signals conversion to wet macular degeneration.

Symptom Terms

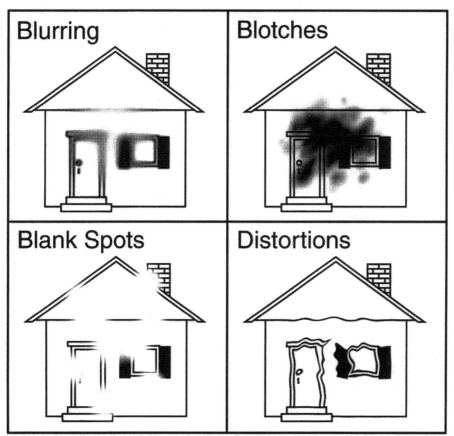

Blurring

Blotches

Blank Spots

Distortions

Wet Macular Degeneration

   Wet macular degeneration usually starts with distortion in the central field of vision and commonly progresses rapidly over a period of days or weeks. Straight lines appear wavy. The edges of buildings may look wavy or twisted. In some cases wet macular degeneration progresses over a period of months.

Many patients report seeing blank spots in the center of their visual field. Or, they may have blurred vision or an increased blurring of their vision, which they may attribute to needing new glasses. Sometimes, due to the blurring, they may think they have cataracts.

Another commonly described symptom is what appears to be a central smudge, like an oily fingerprint, which interferes with central vision. In some cases it is so bothersome that patients have an urge to "wipe it away."

Difficulty Describing Symptoms

Many patients have difficulty describing their symptoms accurately. Some individuals have described their impaired central vision as "a smudge," "ink on a blotter," "a screen in front of my eye," or "my vision is blotted out." Over time, these "spots" can enlarge, effectively blotting out ever-larger sections of central vision.

Any visual changes should be immediately communicated to a doctor for assessment. Patients should talk with their doctors, with the goal of coming up with a common language to describe symptoms. It is more effective to use just a handful of terms, such as the ones suggested in the next paragraph.

One term commonly used to describe visual changes is *blurring*. Here, one may notice that edges of buildings are less distinct—the edges lose their definition. The second term is *blotches*, in which gray or black stains appear in a person's view, obstructing the lines on the Amsler Grid at some points. The third term, *blank spots*, refers to some areas on the grid that disappear from view. The final term is *distortion*, in which lines appear wavy. By having a common vocabulary, patients and doctors will

Amsler Grid

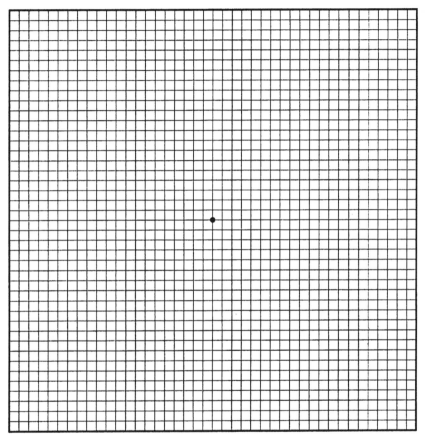

be communicating exactly the kind of information needed to help make informed treatment decisions. Anyone over age 50 who experiences these symptoms should arrange for an immediate eye exam.

One patient, a 63-year-old man named Frank, allowed himself to be talked out of seeing an ophthalmologist by his well-meaning family and friends. The blurring he saw in the center of his field of vision in his right eye was just "old age" creeping in, his friends joked at his weekly bowling league. He tried eyedrops, resting his eyes, even a new vitamin supplement that was touted to help improve vision. Nothing worked. By the time he was examined by an ophthalmologist several weeks later, a hemorrhage had permanently damaged his vision.

Self-Tests for Detecting Early Symptoms

Using the Amsler Grid

Fortunately, there are some simple and easy-to-use methods to detect symptoms of macular degeneration. Perhaps the best way to detect early symptoms, such as distortions and blank spots, is to regularly use the *Amsler Grid*. Basically, the Amsler Grid is like a sheet of graph paper with a dot in the center. To use it, hold the grid about fourteen inches from your eyes. Reading glasses or bifocals should be kept on while using it.

Then gently cover one eye with the palm of the free hand, and focus on the central dot in the middle of the grid. Without moving your eye off the central dot, determine if any lines anywhere on the grid appear distorted or fade or disappear. After opening the closed eye for a few seconds to let it adjust, repeat the test for the second eye.

Naturally, if one eye already has poor vision, that eye will be harder to test using the Amsler Grid. A good technique in this circumstance is to carefully draw the current areas of distortion and blurring on the Amsler Grid so that any future changes can be readily detected. This also reinforces the importance of getting regular eye exams, especially if a person suspects there is another problem in the eye with poor vision.

In some patients, the position of the blank spot that they record on the grid may slowly move over a period of time. In other cases, the shape of the blank spots may change somewhat. That movement is called *remodeling.* Even though remodeling may not indicate that macular degeneration is progressing, patients should be sure to record those changes and report them immediately to a doctor. Only a doctor can properly evaluate remodeling patterns.

People over age 50 are encouraged to use the Amsler Grid every day, whether or not they presently have macular degeneration. If any changes whatsoever are noted—however minor—they should be brought to the attention of an eye doctor. It is a good idea to record on paper as much detail about the symptoms as possible. Symptoms of macular degeneration can cause quite a bit of anxiety, and unless they are written down, crucial details may be forgotten by the time the patient talks to a physician.

Testing Distance Vision

Another good method for detecting the early warning signs of macular degeneration is to test distance vision. There are many visual cues in the environment that can be used to test for symptoms of macular degeneration. Tall buildings, for example, offer straight lines, as do lampposts, telephone poles, and highway signs. Stare at a fixed spot in the distance, close and cover one eye, and see if any of the straight-line cues appear distorted or wavy, or if there are blank spots. Then, repeat with the other eye.

Testing Medium-Range Distance Indoors

You can test your eyes indoors using the line found in corners, where two walls or a wall and ceiling meet, or along the edge of a window. The edges of doors are another good place to look. Only one eye at a time should be tested.

Original handcrafted plastered walls and ceilings in very old homes may have joints with wavy lines, so do not rely on them to test for visual distortion. Instead, use window frames or other areas with known straight lines.

Reading offers another testing opportunity. Stare at a central point on this page, then cover one eye and see if any of the printed lines appear wavy or distorted. Then repeat for the other eye. Look along the edge of the page and check to see if it appears straight. Check for blank spots.

Wavy lines on a printed page prompt many elderly patients to visit their doctors. These patients are often avid readers and suddenly notice they are distracted by lines of print that are out of alignment. Again, catching a problem early may save one's sight.

Test Each Eye Individually

Each eye should be checked individually when using the Amsler Grid or any other self-test for early signs of macular degeneration. There are a couple of reasons for this.

Dominant Eye

In most people one eye is dominant, even though they are not aware of it. The dominant eye is the eye that does most of the looking and will be the eye of choice when that person looks through a camera or telescope. The vision in both eyes may be perfectly fine, but one eye may be preferred in terms of its wiring to the brain.

Amblyopia

During development (until age 8), if both eyes are not used equally, one eye will become stronger. Even with only a small amount of misalignment, the eye that is not used can permanently lose its ability to see, becoming what is called *amblyopic.* In other cases, amblyopia may be caused by a nearsighted or farsighted eye in a young child that caused a blurred image, forcing the other eye to dominate. If the vision is not corrected while the child is still young, permanent loss of vision results. An amblyopic eye typically has 20/50 to 20/200 vision, even with glasses, because the nerves have never developed properly. This is a more severe condition than mere eye dominance. Many people have amblyopia. If each eye is not checked individually, the development of macular degeneration in a nondominant or amblyopic eye could be missed until it is too late.

Testing to Find Your Dominant Eye

To determine which eye is dominant, look at a small object from across a room. Make a little round circle with the thumbs and forefingers of both hands placed together and held out in front. With both eyes open, aim that circle at the small object. Now, close one eye and then the other eye. With one eye open, the circle will still be on the small object. With the other eye open, the circle will look as if it jumped off the object. Whichever eye stays on the object is the dominant eye.

A person needs to be especially vigilant in testing the nondominant eye because the dominant eye will often mask its symptoms.

Tips for Better Testing

Make no mistake about it. As simple as these self-tests may seem, they can detect macular degeneration months earlier than it might otherwise be detected. Macular degeneration can progress very rapidly, so even a few weeks' difference in detecting it can make it dramatically more difficult to treat. Keep the following tips in mind:

- Make sure family members and friends understand the importance of self-testing and remind each other to self-test regularly.
- Conduct the self-tests at about the same time every day, so that it becomes part of a daily routine.
- Keep the Amsler Grid easily accessible. Post it on the refrigerator door, next to the bathroom mirror, or at the computer monitor.
- Be sure to schedule an annual eye exam, not to take the place of self-testing but to add another layer of medical assurance. Scheduling exams near annual events like a birthday helps remind people that their eye exam is due.

Symptoms of Macular Degeneration Progressing

Once it begins, macular degeneration can progress quickly or slowly, through a range of symptoms. The retina has a limited number of ways it can signal changes to the brain. It has no pain fibers, so it cannot send a pain message to indicate something is wrong. So, when something happens to the retina, it sends a signal—typically flashes of light.

These flashes of light can be an important telltale sign of changes in the retina related to macular degeneration. For a patient with macular degeneration, flashes of light may indicate a worsening of the condition, such as increased fluid leakage, hemorrhage, or scarring. For people unsure of whether they have macular degeneration, flashes of light may be an early warning sign.

On the other hand, flashes of light sometimes mean that fluid under the retina is decreasing, that a hemorrhage is being reabsorbed, or that a scar is being changed and stabilized by the body. Since flashes of light signal that changes are occurring, they should trigger an immediate visit to an eye care specialist. Many flashes of light may be a sign of *retinal detachment*, an extremely serious situation, in which the retina becomes detached from the wall of the eye.

Flashes of light are difficult to interpret and typically are not the first sign one has of macular degeneration. Usually flashes occur later on in the progression of the disease.

In some cases, patients may see extremely sharp images, even though they lost their central vision due to macular degeneration many years before. These "phantom" images typically occur only after the patient has had macular degeneration for years. Patients who have no central vision may report seeing faces. Although the faces may not be familiar, they still look very real. More often than not, these phantom images occur in patients with longstanding loss of central vision in both eyes.

In other cases, phantom images will appear in the form of patterns, even elaborate scenes of flowers, trees, or landscapes. Some people will see these images for minutes, while for others the images will appear fleetingly. They can be in color or black and white.

These phantom images can be quite frightening, especially when they first appear. Many patients worry that these images may be symptoms of a brain problem. While phantom images are quite common, especially if both eyes are involved, they should be reported to a specialist.

3

Getting a Diagnosis

To correctly diagnose macular degeneration a doctor will first listen to the patient's description of symptoms, then conduct a comprehensive eye examination. That examination tells the physician whether and to what extent macular degeneration is present. If the disease is present, the physician will set up a management program.

The Eye Examination

The first step in piecing together the clues leading to a diagnosis is to give the patient a thorough eye examination. When an eye doctor inspects a patient's eyes, the first things checked are vital signs, listed below.

Visual Acuity

Visual acuity is measured on an eye chart, using numbers such as 20/20, 20/50, or 20/200. Visual acuity of 20/20 is considered the norm for a healthy person. Visual acuity of 20/50 indicates that an object or letter on an eye chart that should be discernible from 50 feet must be brought to 20 feet in front of the person in order to be identified. Similarly, visual acuity of 20/200 indicates that an object or letter that should be discernible from 200 feet must be brought to 20 feet in front of the person in order to be identified.

Since visual acuity measures central vision, it is important in tests of macular degeneration. Many of the older eye charts do not use equal steps of vision. The newer Early Treatment Diabetic Retinopathy Study (ETDRS) chart, named after a large clinical study performed in the United States on patients with diabetes, does progress in equal increments and thereby allows a better assessment of changes in vision.

Often, by having the patient look through a single pinhole or multiple pinholes, the physician can get an estimate of the best vision that could be achieved if eyeglass lenses were more optimal. This is an easy and useful method to estimate whether a change in glasses would be beneficial.

Another method ophthalmologists use is to put different lenses in front of the patient's eye in order to determine which lenses would improve vision most. The results of this test are compared with the lenses currently being worn, if any. This process is called *refraction*. In the past, these procedures were all performed manually. However, today there are computerized systems that can usually help a doctor get an excellent approximation automatically. The doctor can then focus his or her skills on the more important task of fine-tuning the lenses.

Eye Pressure

A doctor will also test the pressure inside the eye. This test is important to screen for *glaucoma*, a condition causing damage to the optic nerve as the result of pressure in the eye, and other eye health problems. Eye pressure is measured with a tiny instrument that pushes on the eye to determine how hard or soft it is. The test is similar in some ways to testing the pressure in a bicycle tire by pressing on the tire. A combination of a numbing eyedrop and the minimal pressure applied by the measuring instrument make this test painless.

Visual Field

Visual field testing primarily measures peripheral vision. The test is performed by having a person look at a small central point while variously sized objects are projected at various locations away from the center. The individual being tested is asked to signal as soon as these objects become visible.

Eye and General Medical History

Like detectives, eye doctors try to gather all the necessary information and clues to lead to a correct diagnosis so that they may develop an effective treatment plan. To accomplish this, they will gather information on the history of the present illness, including a detailed history of all aspects of the patient's current eye problem(s). They will also ask about the patient's past ocular history, along with a general medical history, including any allergies and any history of smoking or alcohol use. Doctors will ask about medications currently being taken and at some point will systematically collect information about all other potential health problems. Part of the medical history will also include a family medical history.

Examination of the Front of the Eye

The front of the eye largely contains those elements that focus the image on the retina, namely the cornea, iris, and lens.

- **Range of Movement**: The doctor will check whether the eyes move freely and are in alignment. The alignment is very important in order to avoid *double vision*, seeing two of an object.

- **Eyelids**: The eyelids are checked for any evidence of infection or malfunction.

- **Tear Film**: This is a type of fluid, or tear, that bathes and lubricates the cornea of the eyeball. As we age the tear film often becomes less capable of keeping the surface of the eye properly lubricated. This is called *dry eye* but has no relationship to *dry* macular degeneration. Dry eye is often treated with artificial teardrops. Other treatments are available if these drops are not sufficient to address the symptoms. The way the tear film spreads over the surface of an eye can often suggest whether that eye will have symptoms of dryness.

- **Conjunctiva**: A mucus membrane that lines the inside of the eyelids and extends over the front of the white part of the eye. Inflammation can often cause redness. Redness or hemorrhage of the conjunctiva usually has no relationship to what is going on within the retina. However, excessive inflammation can be a sign of infection or allergy.

- **Cornea**: The cornea is the clear front surface of the eye. It is responsible for most of the eye's focusing power. When examining the cornea, the physician will look for evidence of irritation, inflammation, and infection.

- **Anterior Chamber**: The anterior chamber is the clear, fluid-filled space separating the cornea and iris. Signs of inflammation, infection, or hemorrhage can sometimes be early warning signals of a problem with the overall health of the eye.

- **Iris**: The iris is the portion of the eye that gives it color (blue, hazel, brown). The iris controls the size of the pupil, enlarging to allow more light to enter in low-light situations and constricting to reduce the light entering in bright-light situations. Problems of the iris are relatively rare but can occur in certain situations, including diabetic eye problems and certain types of inflammation.

- **Lens**: Besides the cornea, the other main component for focusing images is the lens. A clouding of the lens is called a *cataract.* If a cataract becomes cloudy enough to significantly impair vision, it can be removed and replaced with an artificial lens called an *implant.* Examination of the lens is performed to determine if a cataract is present and to judge its severity.

Examination of the Back of the Eye

The back of the eye is the crucial portion of the exam for evaluating macular degeneration. However, doctors do not actually view the back of the eye. Instead, they view the retina by looking through the pupil, much like looking through a peephole in a door. A lens is used to magnify the doctor's field of view.

- **Vitreous**: This clear, gel-like, central portion of the eye can, on rare occasion, contain some blood leaking from under the retina in patients with macular degeneration.

- **Peripheral Retina**: A number of eye disorders involve the peripheral retina. While this area is generally not affected by macular degeneration, the doctor will examine it to be sure other eye disorders are not involved.

- **Central Retina or Macula**: Several components of the central retina or macula are involved when macular degeneration occurs. Therefore, a retinal specialist will devote a great deal of attention to this part of the exam. In particular, the physician will look for the following conditions to confirm a diagnosis of dry or wet macular degeneration.

Signs of Dry Macular Degeneration

- **Drusen**: If larger drusen with indistinct borders are present, it alerts the physician to the possibility that macular degeneration has already begun or may be progressing; it also raises the patient's risk of getting wet macular degeneration.

- **Pigment**: Flecks of brown or black indicate changes in the cells that separate the retina from its underlying blood vessels. The presence of pigment raises the risk of getting macular degeneration and serves to alert the physician to a diagnosis of macular degeneration.

- **Central Atrophy or Other Atrophy in the Macula**: *Atrophy* is a thinning of the retina that may occur as part of dry macular degeneration. It can signal a loss of retinal tissue that may contribute to vision loss.

Signs of Wet Macular Degeneration

The signs of wet macular degeneration are more definitive.

- **Subretinal Fluid**: Fluid that has accumulated under the retina is a telltale sign of macular degeneration.

- **Subretinal Blood**: Blood accumulating under the retina is another sign of macular degeneration.

- **Lipids**: The presence of lipids, fatty deposits, in the blood indicates prolonged wet macular degeneration.

- **Retinal Thickening**: The retina may thicken due to its being saturated with fluids. This may precede the eventual creation of a bubble under the retina and indicates that macular degeneration is present.

Performing an Angiogram

As part of making an accurate diagnosis, a physician may decide to do an *angiogram.* In this procedure, the physician places a special dye into a vein in the patient's arm. When the dye reaches the retina, the physician photographs the eyeball with a special high-speed camera. The information is then processed by a powerful computer, giving the physician a better understanding of the current status of the patient's condition.

Once the diagnosis is complete—the retina assessed for damage and the rate of progression of disease estimated—the physician can determine what treatment options are available for the patient.

Angiography

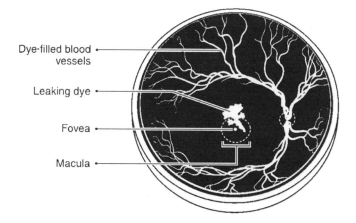

Dye-filled blood vessels

Leaking dye

Fovea

Macula

In this representation of an angiogram, the dye, shown leaking from the blood vessel, indicates development of macular degeneration.

4

Risk Factors for Macular Degeneration

Scientists worldwide are researching what behaviors, foods, genes, and other factors may put people at risk for getting macular degeneration. We now understand some of these factors. In other cases, we have preliminary studies that promise to give us more details on risk factors in the future. As risk factors are discovered, physicians develop ways to better prevent, delay, and treat macular degeneration. By understanding the major risk factors, people can reduce their risk of getting macular degeneration and the damage it does.

Age

One of the unfortunate truths about aging is that it makes us more susceptible to various diseases, including macular degeneration. In fact, age is the greatest risk factor for macular degeneration. Beyond age 55, the chance of getting macular degeneration increases. People over 55, and most especially those over 65, should be vigilant about testing their eyes regularly and treating macular degeneration as early as possible.

Genetics

Despite the many difficulties of conducting genetic research, scientists have determined that genetics does play a role in macular degeneration. For example, macular degeneration is more prevalent among Caucasians, Asians, and Greenlanders than among African-Americans and Hispanics. Similarly, studies of relatives of people with macular degeneration have shown they are three times as likely to have the disease as relatives of people who do not have macular degeneration. Another study has shown that the risk of getting macular degeneration is approximately 19 times higher for a sibling of someone with macular degeneration than for a sibling of someone without the disease.

Studies of identical and fraternal twins provide strong evidence that macular degeneration is genetically determined. Since identical twins are formed from a single sperm and egg, they have the same DNA. Therefore, they should both inherit the same disorders. Fraternal twins, on the other hand, are formed from two separate eggs fertilized by two separate sperm. Theoretically, they should have an inherited disorder at the same rate as non-twin siblings. A large study completed in 1995 proved the case. It showed that in all sets of identical twins both members had macular degeneration, compared with fraternal twins where only 42 percent had macular degeneration in common.

Scientists will not rest until they find the gene or genes responsible for predisposing a person to macular degeneration, that research is going on right now. Recently the gene for a macular disorder related to macular degeneration was found, raising the hope that researchers will be similarly successful with macular degeneration.

While genetic influences are obviously important, they are greatly influenced by some of the other risk factors discussed below. Smoking, for example, may increase a person's odds of getting macular degeneration more than genetic factors. On the flip side, eating lots of green leafy vegetables may reduce a person's risk of getting macular degeneration, even if the genes predisposing that person to the disorder are present.

Smoking

There is good data showing that people who smoke are at a much higher risk for getting macular degeneration than people who do not smoke. One reason is that substances found in cigarettes alter blood flow to the *choroid*, the network of blood vessels under the eye. While the risk of developing macular degeneration is increased for both men and women smokers, the risk is even more pronounced in women.

Dietary Factors

Numerous medical studies seem to reinforce the old saying that "we are what we eat." Evidence seems to be mounting that poor dietary practices increase one's risk of getting macular degeneration. Conversely, eating a healthy diet may decrease one's risk.

To understand why poor nutrition may increase the likelihood of getting macular degeneration, it is useful to know about *free radicals*. Every second of every day, free radicals are being formed in the body as a result of digesting food, converting food to energy, repairing injuries, and in thousands of other biochemical reactions. Free radicals are molecules that are full of energy, waiting to react with other molecules in the body to release some of that energy. If they happen to meet up with a sensitive system within the body, such as our DNA, the genetic code that determines who we are, they can damage it. Such damage contributes to many health disorders, including cancer.

As we have already seen, the cells of the retina are very active, which means that free radicals are constantly being formed there. These free radicals can damage the sensitive light receptors and adjoining cells of the retina and may increase the chance that a person will get macular degeneration.

There are natural systems in the body designed to inactivate free radicals. Difficulties arise when unhealthy eating increases the sheer number of free radicals in the body. Fortunately, certain vitamins and other nutrients found in healthy diets also help to inactivate free radicals.

Sunlight

Medical researchers are still unclear whether and to what degree exposure to sunlight increases one's risk of getting macular degeneration. Laboratory research has shown that *ultraviolet (UV) light* can damage retinal cells. But this laboratory research has not been supported by medical field research. One such classic study involved watermen on the Chesapeake Bay. Watermen spend many hours each day dredging for oysters, catching crabs, or fishing. They are subject not only to harsh sunlight but to light reflected off the water, so we would expect them to be at high risk for developing macular degeneration if sunlight were the culprit that some suspect it to be. However, the study showed no correlation between the men's long periods of exposure to intense sunlight and the development of macular degeneration. But this same study did show that those who wore no eye protection had three times as many cataracts as those who wore sunglasses or a wide-brimmed hat.

Another line of research, again based on animal and laboratory experiments, points to the blue portion of the sun's light spectrum as being the most damaging to the sensitive retinal cells. Sunlight contains the red, orange, yellow, green, blue, indigo, and violet portions of the light spectrum. *Blue light*—namely blue, indigo, and violet—contains the most energy.

Based on these laboratory and animal studies, some scientists believe that UV and blue light together may somehow be involved in the aging of the retina and in causing or worsening macular degeneration. Excessive exposure to intense sunlight can also cause *pterygium*, a scarring of the cornea.

High Blood Pressure

In the past ten years, significant medical studies have shown that people with high blood pressure have a higher incidence of wet macular degeneration and that it progresses faster, when compared to those with normal blood pressure. Another study has shown that people with high blood pressure have a higher incidence of dry macular degeneration. These studies point to the importance of regularly checking blood pressure.

Physicians believe that since macular degeneration is a problem with the outer blood supply to the retina, it makes sense that high blood pressure would affect it negatively. High blood pressure is one of the most thoroughly documented risk factors for both large and small blood vessel diseases. After years and years of blood coursing through the small arteries at high pressure, it is not surprising that it eventually causes some damage.

In a young, healthy person the walls of the arteries have a good deal of stretch to them. As blood pulses through, the stretching action actually reduces the pressure exerted on the walls. However, as we age, the vessels are less apt to stretch properly. Coupled with high blood pressure, the tiny blood vessels of the eye can be more easily damaged in the elderly.

Cardiovascular Disease

Scientists are beginning to believe that cardiovascular disease increases one's risk of macular degeneration.

Arteriosclerosis

For years, medical researchers have worked under the theory that high amounts of fatty substances and cholesterol in the blood-stream promote *arteriosclerosis*, a thickening of the walls of the small blood vessels. In terms of macular degeneration, physicians believed that over a period of decades the blood vessels of the choroid thickened and eventually lead to macular degeneration. In fact, many years ago macular degeneration was known as hardening of the arteries of the choroid.

Unfortunately, we still do not know with certainty whether high levels of fatty substances and cholesterol in the blood contribute to macular degeneration. Some studies have shown this effect, while others have not. No one has been able to come up with a satisfactory explanation for the discrepancies in these studies. However, we do have enough data to show that these substances cause problems in small blood vessels in other parts of the body.

Atherosclerosis

Atherosclerosis is a disease in which fatty deposits and plaques accumulate on the walls of the large blood vessels. These deposits can restrict blood flow and cause changes in the walls of the blood vessels. In 1995, a study conducted in the Netherlands showed that people with plaques in the carotid arteries of the neck had a 4.7 times greater chance of developing macular degeneration than people without plaques.

Similarly, another good study showed that people with high pulse pressure, a further indicator of cardiovascular disease, had a 30 percent increased incidence of macular degeneration and a 25 percent increase in its rate of progression than a control group without high pulse pressure. *Pulse pressure* is the difference between a person's systolic and diastolic blood pressure readings. In other words, if a person's blood pressure is 120 over 80, the pulse pressure is 40.

Diabetes

Increased blood sugar causes abnormalities in the structure and functioning of the choroidal blood vessels, the retinal pigment epithelium, and Bruch's membrane. These abnormalities may increase a person's risk of getting macular degeneration.

Body Weight

Two large medical studies have shown a relationship between being overweight and an increased risk of getting macular degeneration. One large study showed that greater body mass was associated with dry macular degeneration, but not wet macular degeneration. Another large study in Colorado showed that people with a higher waist-hip ratio had a greater incidence of dry macular degeneration than people with a lower ratio. The waist-hip ratio is a measure of fat distribution. As one's waist measurement begins to approach one's hip measurement—the proverbial and much-dreaded "pear" shape—it indicates that fat is being accumulated in the body.

Farsightedness and Nearsightedness

There is mixed evidence that farsightedness and nearsightedness increase a person's risk of getting macular degeneration. Some smaller studies have suggested a relationship between far-sightedness and macular degeneration, but larger follow-up studies have failed to show such a relationship.

Cataracts and Cataract Surgery

Experts disagree over whether having cataracts increases one's chances of getting macular degeneration. No studies have consistently shown that having cataracts increases a person's risk of developing either dry or wet macular degeneration.

One large study showed an increased rate of progression in wet macular degeneration after cataract removal. However, other studies have failed to confirm this finding.

On the surface, it may sound absurd to think that it could be harmful to remove a condition that is causing severe visual loss in a person. However, ophthalmologists believe that the lens, which is removed during cataract surgery, actually protects the retina from the harmful effects of blue light. Without the lens serving as a blue light filter, the cells of the retina are exposed to increased damage, which either promotes dry macular degeneration or increases the rate at which wet macular degeneration progresses.

There may be other reasons why removal of the lens might cause macular degeneration to develop or accelerate. Part of the answer may be in the very act of surgery itself. The lens is attached to the vitreous and when it is removed, it may pull on the delicate macula. In patients who already have wet macular degeneration, this pulling may cause fragile blood vessels to rupture. Also during surgery, the pressure in the eye drops during the minutes it takes for the surgeon to remove the lens. That loss of pressure creates a vacuum effect on the retina, thereby pulling on sensitive capillaries and perhaps causing them to rupture.

Glaucoma

Glaucoma is an eye disorder characterized by an increase of pressure within the eyeball. People with glaucoma are not at any greater risk for developing macular degeneration. No studies show any relationship between glaucoma or the use of eyedrops for glaucoma and the development of macular degeneration.

Assessing Your Risk

A person's risk for losing vision from macular degeneration is a combination of many factors, including family history, general health, nutrition, lifestyle, and current extent of macular degeneration.

The simple self-test here gives patients an opportunity to go to their first doctor's visit already having gathered important information that will aid in their treatment.

Self-Assessment Item	Your Score	Subtotals
Part A		
I am:		
over 55 years old (score **30**)		
over 65 years old (score **35**)		
over 75 years old (score **40**)		
over 85 years old (score **50**)		
I have:		
a parent, brother, or sister who has been diagnosed with macular degeneration (score **10**)		
a cousin, aunt, or uncle who has been diagnosed with macular degeneration (score **5**)		
My total cholesterol level is:		
240 mg/dl or higher (score **10**)		
220-239 mg/dl (score **5**)		
200-219 mg/dl (score **3**)		
175-199 mg/dl (score **1**)		
below 175 mg/dl (score **0**)		
I drink more than 2 to 3 alcoholic drinks per day (score **5**)		
I smoke more than one pack a day (score **15**)		
I smoke less than a pack a day (score **10**)		
I live or work with people who smoke every day (score **5**)		
Generally, I get less than 30 minutes of daily physical activity consistent with my general health (score **5**)		

I have blood or fluid under the retina (score **20**)		
Add Part A	⇨	
Part B		
I check my close vision in each eye daily with an Amsler Grid or similar test (score **20**)		
I check my distance vision in each eye daily (score **20**)		
I have developed a detailed follow-up schedule of exams with my eye care provider (score **20**)		
I drink: one glass of red wine per day (for a male) (score **3**) three glasses of red wine per week (for a female) (score **3**)		
I eat at least one cup of green leafy vegetables per day (score **7**)		
My HDL ("good") cholesterol level is more than 35 mg/dl (score **7**)		
Add Part B	⇨	
Subtract Part B score from Part A score to arrive at your total score	⇨	

How to Interpret the Risk Assessment

The self-assessment can provide only a rough indication of a person's risk for getting macular degeneration. That is because medical science does not yet understand all the variables that lead a person to have macular degeneration that progresses to vision loss. Also uncertain is the exact degree of risk posed by any one factor. The self-assessment can help determine a person's relative risk of having vision impaired by macular degeneration. However, since everyone is unique, consult your eye doctor to more accurately determine risks, prevention strategies, and treatment options.

If the score is:

100 or above	The risk of losing vision from macular degeneration is relatively high.
70-99	The risk of losing vision from macular degeneration is moderately high.
30-69	This is an average risk of losing vision from macular degeneration.
Below 30	The risk of losing vision from macular degeneration is low.

5

Reducing the Risk of Macular Degeneration

It is important to be in good health for our eyes to function properly and to lessen our risk of developing macular degeneration. By eating properly, avoiding risky health behaviors, and exercising regularly, our bodies will serve us well and we reduce the odds of getting a range of diseases. Maintaining that balance will also go a long way toward preventing macular degeneration and the difficulties it causes.

Keep Coronary Arteries Healthy

As we have seen, people who have coronary artery disease appear to be at greater risk of getting macular degeneration. Fortunately, scientists know a good deal about the causes, risk factors, and prevention of coronary artery disease. As the risk of getting coronary artery disease is reduced, the risk of getting or worsening macular degeneration may also be reduced. The following are ways to reduce the risk of getting coronary artery disease.

Stop Smoking

One important action a person can take to reduce the risk of coronary artery disease is to stop smoking. Smoking shortens life and increases the risk of getting many diseases, including macular degeneration. Research has shown that tobacco may actually interfere with the body's absorption of lutein, which plays a central role in protecting the retina. Smokers tend to have lower blood levels of lutein than do nonsmokers. That may be one reason why smokers have higher rates of macular degeneration.

Quitting smoking is very difficult. Nonetheless, many programs are now available to quit smoking, from the use of nicotine patches to behavior modification programs to group therapy. It may take several attempts to finally quit, but it is well worth the effort. In any event, quitting significantly reduces a person's risk of getting macular degeneration.

Control Blood Cholesterol

Cholesterol comes only from animal products—meat, dairy, or eggs. Fruits, vegetables, vegetable oils, grains, nuts, and seeds do not contain any cholesterol. There are two main types of cholesterol. "Good" cholesterol is known as *HDL*, or *high-density lipids.* "Bad" cholesterol is known as *LDL*, or *low-density lipids.* (To help you remember that LDL is the bad cholesterol, think of the *L* as standing for "lousy.")

The body already makes all the cholesterol it needs. That is why people should limit their daily intake of cholesterol to no more than 300 milligrams a day, although considerably less would be even better. The key to better heart health is to keep one's blood cholesterol level to 240 milligrams or less.

People with a total cholesterol level above 240 should speak with a doctor about a regimen to lower it. In some cases, raising the HDL level (by exercising, for example) may suffice. In other cases, high cholesterol levels may need to be lowered with medication. No matter what the treatment, it is critical to lower high levels of cholesterol to prevent coronary artery disease.

Control High Blood Pressure

High blood pressure itself, even without accompanying coronary artery disease, may increase a person's risk for both dry and wet macular degeneration. However, the good news is that there are many ways to control high blood pressure. Even with those factors that cannot be controlled, such as race or genetic makeup, there are ways to monitor and reduce the severity of the disease.

One way to reduce high blood pressure is to limit the intake of salt. Although there has been contradictory evidence about the role of salt in high blood pressure, present knowledge still weighs in on the side of being prudent about salt intake, especially for those who already have high blood pressure. Just 1¼ teaspoons of table salt contains 2,400 milligrams.

Medical research has also shown that many responses to stress raise blood pressure. A person who lives a life in which stress is not properly managed should consider developing a stress management plan. Some of the meditation techniques now taught, when practiced regularly, help to reduce stress.

Since high blood pressure has few, if any, noticeable symptoms, the importance of regular monitoring cannot be emphasized enough. People with high blood pressure should be sure their physician is aware of all their risk factors so that a suitable monitoring program can be designed.

Aim for Ideal Body Weight

People who are well above the ideal body weight for their height are at far greater risk of developing coronary artery disease and high blood pressure than those who are at or slightly below ideal body weight. Anyone more than 10 percent above ideal body weight should speak with a physician about options for getting back to ideal weight. The most effective programs combine diet, good nutrition, and exercise. Fad diets rarely work and often result in the seesaw weight swings that plague so many people throughout their lives. The most effective weight loss and maintenance program is one that changes a person's behaviors and lifestyle.

Control Diabetes

An unfortunate reality of diabetes is that it increases the risk of developing cardiovascular disease, even if glucose levels are well controlled. An annual physical examination should include a test for diabetes, especially if a person is over 50. People who already have diabetes must be vigilant about controlling the disease. Working with a healthcare provider, diabetics should try to control any other risk factors they can. The actual role of diabetes in the development of macular degeneration is not clear. However, diabetes can exacerbate cardiovascular disease and high blood pressure, which in turn can affect macular degeneration.

Exercise Regularly

Regular exercise decreases the risk of coronary artery disease and high blood pressure. But exercise also improves general health and the health of the entire circulatory system. The better the health of the circulatory system, the lower is one's risk of developing macular degeneration.

Exercise does not have to mean going to a fancy, expensive gym. A good workout could be a brisk thirty-minute walk, so long as it puts a certain demand on the heart and lungs. Exactly what that demand is depends on many factors, such as age, level of fitness at the beginning of the exercise program, and the individual's exercise goals. That is why it is best to consult with a physician before beginning a program. There are many fitness professionals available for a consult after a doctor gives the okay to begin. A good idea is to join a gym, even if it is only for a special introductory program for a few months, since memberships usually include an initial consult and instruction on how to warm up and do various exercises properly.

Since macular degeneration is mostly a disease of people older than 50, and most usually over 65, older patients may need to be counseled on the value of exercise. There is no question that exercise at any age is helpful. The problem is that some patients view exercise in unrealistic terms. A seventy-year-old man cannot compare his exercise program to that of a much younger man.

An effective exercise program is based on age, physical condition, medical conditions, and personal goals. The key is to begin and then to continue on a regular basis. Today, there are wonderful walking programs for seniors available in malls. There are aquatic exercise programs for people with arthritis. And there are even limbering programs for octogenarians! Whatever one's age or level of fitness, an assessment by a physician can help one begin and stay on an exercise program.

Use Alcohol in Moderation

In healthy adults without coronary artery disease or high blood pressure, recent medical research suggests that moderate alcohol consumption—one glass (4 fluid ounces) of red wine per day for men or three glasses of red wine a week for women—may actually offer some protection from macular degeneration.

However, excessive alcohol use increases a person's risk of high blood pressure and subsequent coronary artery disease. That, in turn, increases one's risk of macular degeneration. That is why alcohol must be consumed in moderation.

Nutritious Eating

Some of the most exciting research on macular degeneration taking place today is in the area of nutrition. Unfortunately, what the general public has heard about this research is largely biased and sensational, touting one or another of a long list of vitamins and minerals as miracle cures for macular degeneration. Based on what scientists know today about good nutrition generally, and the nutrition of the eye in particular, there are sound dietary practices that are likely to increase the health of the eye as well as overall health and well-being. While the role of diet in helping to prevent macular degeneration is not yet proven, early research is promising enough for people to use wise nutritional practices as part of a comprehensive plan to reduce their risk.

Eat Green Leafy Vegetables

Green leafy vegetables are nature's vitamin and mineral factories. Initial studies have shown that green leafy vegetables do offer some protection from macular degeneration. But researchers do not know for sure exactly how much of these vegetables we need to eat to get the maximum protective effect. Studies to determine this are taking place right now. However, preliminary results are encouraging enough that everyone concerned about their eyes should eat at least one serving (1 cup) of green leafy vegetables every day.

Green leafy vegetables are high in two strange-sounding vitamins: *lutein* (loo-tee-in) and *zeaxanthin* (zee-a-zan-thin), both of which are *carotenoids*, a type of vitamin. It is important to know that lutein and zeaxanthin supplements sold by vitamin companies may turn out to be more hype than reality. Why? Medical research makes no claim that lutein (or zeaxanthin) is causing the protective effects. Researchers have only found that regularly eating green leafy vegetables reduces a person's risk of getting macular degeneration. It may be that lutein plays a big role. Or it may be that lutein, combined with some of the other hundreds of nutrients in green leafy vegetables, is responsible for protecting our eyes. It might even be true that it is not lutein at all, but some other compound in green leafy vegetables that is responsible for the beneficial effects. The truth will not be known until further research is conducted.

Vegetables that are high in lutein and zeaxanthin include kale, spinach, turnip and collard greens, romaine lettuce, and broccoli. Vegetables and fruits of other colors are also high in lutein and zeaxanthin. Corn, orange peppers, red grapes, kiwi fruit, oranges, and zucchini are good examples. Eggs contain both lutein and zeaxanthin, according to some British researchers. And, speaking of eggs, we now know that while they boost bad cholesterol, they also boost good cholesterol, which is needed to rid the body of bad cholesterol. So, the judicious use of eggs seems prudent.

Limit Fats and Choose Them Wisely

The American Heart Association recommends limiting daily fat intake to a *maximum* of 30 percent of total daily calories. That means a 50-year-old woman eating a 2,200-calorie diet should eat no more than 70 grams of fat a day, not an easy task in our country today. Fast foods and commercial snacks can quickly surpass that limit.

Making the matter even more difficult is that people tend to focus on that 30 percent figure and somehow forget that it is a maximum. Many nutritionists say that a healthier total fat intake would be 20 percent of total calories, which translates to approximately 50 grams of fat for someone eating 2,200 calories a day.

Restrict Intake of Saturated Fats

Whether a person chooses 20 percent or 30 percent for total fat intake, or somewhere in between, *saturated fats* should be severely limited. The data are clear that high levels of saturated fats and cholesterol in the bloodstream can lead to heart disease and may possibly lead to increased risk of macular degeneration. The American Heart Association recommends that saturated fats be limited to a maximum of 10 percent of your total daily calories.

Saturated fats come from red meats and from certain plants, such as the coconut and palm. Unfortunately, cocoa butter, a prime ingredient of chocolate, is high in saturated fats. In our society, it is difficult to limit one's intake of saturated fats. That is because we eat far more red meats than we should, more in fact than almost any other country. We also tend to eat desserts and snacks, which are typically made with oils high in saturated fats.

Even when we cook at home we tend to use too much butter, another culprit implicated in macular degeneration. Butter not only contains saturated fats, but also cholesterol, another possible health threat when eaten in large amounts. One tablespoon of butter contains a little more than 7 grams of saturated fats.

How Much Fat?

Want to figure out what your fat intake should be? Start with the ideal number of calories that you should be eating that day. Then divide that number by 30 to get the maximum grams of fat. For example, a 2,200-calorie diet calls for a maximum of 73 grams of fat for someone wishing to stay at the 30 percent total calories from fat level (or, better yet, 50 grams if aiming for a heart-healthier 20 percent total calories from fat).

Limit Use of Polyunsaturated Fats

Vegetable oils from plants such as safflower, sesame, sunflower, corn, and soybeans are *polyunsaturated*. These are better for our health, since they help the body get rid of newly formed cholesterol. However, they are still fats and should be limited to about 10 percent of total calorie intake, or a total of 5 to 7 grams a day.

Use Monounsaturated Fats

Monounsaturated oils may actually help to reduce cholesterol level, so long as total daily fat intake is relatively low. These oils include canola and olive oils. Monounsaturated fats should represent 10 to 15 percent of your total daily calories.

Prepare Foods in Healthful Ways

Nutritionists suggest that food preparation significantly affects our health. It takes very little fat to quickly add up to the daily maximum. Just one piece of deep-fried chicken could easily soak up more than the daily maximum of fat. Nutritionists recommend these food preparation tips:

- Steam vegetables using a dash of spices to permeate them with flavor.

- Sauté vegetables in a very small amount of canola or olive oil. While sautéing, add small amounts of liquids, such as red wine or vegetable stock, to reduce your need for oil and to add flavor.
- Try broiling vegetables, fish, and other meats, using low-fat marinades for zest.
- Poached fish needs no oils. Try poaching in aluminum foil with scallions, red wine, and spices.
- Bake potatoes instead of frying them. When frying, use canola or olive oil lightly in a pan. Never deep-fry potatoes.
- Try nonfat salad dressings and toppings on baked potatoes.
- When making soups that contain meats or fat, refrigerate before serving and skim off all the fat that floats to the top.
- When frying ground beef for a recipe, empty the pan, blot the fat from the meat and the pan, and return the meat to the pan to continue with the recipe.
- Remove all skin from chicken before cooking.
- Gradually change from whole milk to lower-fat milks.
- Eat less red meat, choose leaner cuts of meat, and trim off as much fat as possible. Organ meats (liver, brain, heart) are especially high in cholesterol, so cut way back on them.

Try Soy

The bland nature of soy has been a turnoff to American palates. But bland soy is a thing of the past, as food manufacturers have flocked to its healthy benefits.

A study reported in the *New England Journal of Medicine* several years ago showed that when people substitute soy for animal products, the cholesterol levels in their bloodstream fall by as much as 20 percent. Soy is also high in protein and naturally low in fat. Grocery stores now sell soy burgers, bacon and sausage substitutes, and a host of other products made of soy.

Follow the Food Guidelines

The revised food guidelines from the U.S. Department of Agriculture are a step in the right direction. The Department still has a way to go to bring the guidelines in sync with current nutrition research, but the latest food guidelines are a solid start. They represent a significant departure from the past.

The most important point of the new guidelines is that we should all be eating *most* of our calories in the form of grain products, vegetables, and fruits. That makes sense for a number of reasons. First, these foods contain lots of vitamins, minerals, complex carbohydrates, and other substances that are key to good health. Second, they are generally low in fat. Third, in study after study, their consumption has been associated with a significantly lower risk of many chronic diseases. Fourth, they do not contain any cholesterol. Finally, they are loaded with fiber, which is beneficial to the healthy functioning of our bowels.

The body must be balanced for all systems to function at peak efficiency. That is especially true of our eyes. The eyes are extremely complex organs, placing proportionately large demands on the body's resources. To function well, we must nourish our bodies properly.

As if on cue, the global economy brings us fresh fruit and vegetables year-round. Supermarkets carry a wider variety of fruits, vegetables, and grains than ever before. Years ago, few

Americans had ever heard of quinoa, a South American grain. Now it is one of many new, nutritious grains we eat.

The key to eating a well-balanced, varied diet high in fruits, vegetables, and grains is the Food Guide Pyramid. Weekly menus should be planned around it.

Eat Appropriate Quantities

Eating right is a combination of common sense and good science. A diet that is varied and balanced among the food groups would be a good start. However, while many Americans think they know what a balanced diet is, their eating habits do not necessarily reflect that knowledge.

Eating a balanced diet does not mean giving equal treatment to all foods regarding volume and weight. A serving of salad, for example, should occupy a far larger space on the dinner plate

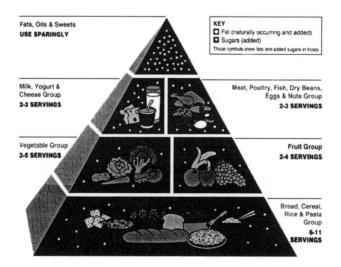

than a serving of meat. Most healthful diets call for a serving portion of meat or fish to be three ounces. That is approximately the space occupied by an adult's palm, *not* including any part of the fingers.

Good food balance does mean that many different foods and food groups should be represented in daily and weekly meals. But attention must be paid to the appropriate quantity for each food group. Notice that the Food Guide Pyramid provides ranges. In the grains and pasta group, the pyramid shows a range of 6 to 11 servings per day. For a woman with a sedentary lifestyle or an older senior, 6 servings a day is enough. Active people need more servings. In general, men would tend to eat the higher number of servings, while women would tend to eat fewer servings. Of course, that is dependent on one's level of activity and other factors. Don't be put off by the 6 to 11 servings a day of grains, cereals, and bread. Most of us, for example, would eat at least a cup of pasta at dinner, which is considered two servings. Also, the way the Food Guide Pyramid was designed, eating the minimum number of servings suggested adds up to approximately 1,600 calories a day, depending on how the foods are prepared.

Be a Cautious Consumer

Astonishing claims are made that mega doses of certain vitamins or minerals will prevent macular degeneration. Unfortunately, no studies accurately support these claims, and they have absolutely no proven role in reversing the effects of macular degeneration.

For vegetarians, the use of supplements is dependent on many factors, such as whether dairy products are eaten, the age, and even the sex of the person. Vegetarians should consult with

Serving Size Examples

Grain Products Group (bread, cereal, rice, and pasta)
1 slice of bread
1 ounce of ready-to-eat cereal
1/2 cup of cooked cereal, rice, or pasta

Vegetable Group
1 cup of raw leafy vegetables
1/2 cup of other vegetables—cooked or chopped raw
3/4 cup of vegetable juice

Fruit Group
1 medium apple, banana, or orange
1/2 cup of chopped, cooked, or canned fruit
3/4 cup of fruit juice

Milk Group (milk, yogurt, and cheese)
1 cup of milk or yogurt
1 1/2 ounces of natural cheese
2 ounces of processed cheese

Meat and Beans Group (meat, poultry, fish, dry beans, eggs, and nuts)

2-3 ounces of cooked lean meat, poultry, or fish
1/2 cup of cooked dry beans or 1 egg counts as 1 ounce of lean meat
2 tablespoons of peanut butter or 1/3 cup of nuts counts as 1 ounce of meat

their physicians or a competent nutritionist before taking supplements.

Many ophthalmologists are concerned about the possibility of damage from high doses of supplements. Before taking any supplements, consult with a physician.

Consumers should be particularly wary of taking large doses of the supplements listed below.

Zinc: Important, but No Miracle Cure

Zinc is probably the most touted substance for the prevention of macular degeneration. A potent antioxidant, it inactivates free radicals. Although zinc is the second most abundant trace element in the body, it is *the* most abundant trace element in the tissues of the eye.

In one reputable study, people with macular degeneration who were given zinc had less visual loss than a control group that was given placebos. Unfortunately, the people that the researchers studied were from a small geographic area in Utah. The study group's social and religious customs, the soil they grew their foods in, and the water they drank were not typical of the general population. Also, due to intermarriage, there was less genetic variability in this group. So, the results are still inconclusive.

Too much zinc can cause a certain type of anemia and can lower the blood levels of the good type of cholesterol, two potentially serious side effects that could be life threatening. High levels of zinc may also accelerate osteoporosis.

No follow-up studies have shown zinc to be the miracle cure for macular degeneration. In fact, a larger study is currently being conducted. However, results will probably not be known for many years.

The U.S. Recommended Dietary Allowance (USRDA) for zinc is 12 milligrams a day for women 19 to 50 years of age. Men require 15 milligrams a day. The best sources of zinc are lean red meats, poultry, and certain shellfish, such as oysters. Meat and dairy products provide approximately 60 percent of the zinc in the typical American diet. Grain products provide about 17 percent.

However, it is often difficult for some people to get enough zinc from their diet. Vegetarians, for example, do not eat meats. Some of the substances in whole grains and the fiber in some plant foods actually interfere with the body's ability to absorb zinc. Zinc deficiency is most common in seniors because they tend to eat fewer zinc-rich foods as they age and their ability to absorb zinc may decline naturally.

People should get as much zinc as possible from foods that are naturally high in the mineral and not depend on supplements. However, if their lifestyles or a vegetarian diet do not allow for adequate amounts of zinc, people should take a simple multivitamin containing no more than the USRDA for this essential mineral.

Vitamins C and E: The Jury Is Still Out

Vitamin C is perhaps the best known of the antioxidants. However, to date there is no proof that high levels of vitamin C prevent macular degeneration or slow its progression.

Likewise, numerous studies have been done on the effects of vitamin E on macular degeneration. Unfortunately, none of them have shown clear results. Some show that vitamin E is effective in preventing some vision loss, while others show no such effect. Again, ongoing studies should provide us with more definitive answers in the future.

Gingko and Bilberry: No Cure

Gingko and *bilberry* are derived from plants. Some have suggested that these substances can help prevent macular degeneration. Unfortunately, there is no evidence that this is true.

On the other hand, these herbal supplements will probably do no harm if taken in moderation. But, taking them should not delay someone seeking expert medical attention. Delaying treatment for macular degeneration is foolish and may result in significant visual loss.

Wear Protective Eyewear

There is a great deal of hype in magazines and on web sites about how sunglasses can prevent macular degeneration. Unfortunately, some of this information is based on preliminary data or unsubstantiated claims.

Although studies of the effects of light on human retinal cells are ongoing, it makes good sense to wear sunglasses anytime a person is outdoors, even on cloudy days. The ultra-violet (UV) portion of sunlight readily passes through clouds and is potentially as damaging to the eye as direct sunlight.

In fact, it is probably wise to protect the eyes against any intense light because of the possibility that light energy might damage sensitive retinal cells. We already know for certain that excessive exposure to intense sunlight can cause pterygium, a scarring of the cornea. People who already have macular degeneration should be vigilant about protecting their remaining sight.

Research also shows that wearing a hat reduces the eyes' exposure to harmful sunlight by approximately half. So, a good line of defense is to always wear both a wide-brimmed hat and sunglasses when outdoors.

Select Quality Sunglasses

It's important to choose good quality sunglasses that will help protect your eyes. However, note that high price does not always mean high quality. Sunglasses have become a fashion accessory in recent years. Prepare to pay a premium for some of the highest-demand brands. But, in many cases, the same quality lenses are available for far less. Look for a similar product without the high-fashion label. The appendix lists some of the major manufacturers of good quality, high-tech sunglasses.

Get Total UV Protection

Shop for sunglasses at a reputable store that provides reliable and complete information. Currently there is no uniform labeling standard for sunglasses. For example, sunglasses labeled as "UV absorbing" may absorb most UV-B light, but not much UV-A light.

Sunglasses should offer 100 percent UV protection for both UV-A and UV-B. The lenses should block out all light under 400 nanometers in wavelength. Lenses designated as having a "UV400 coating" or "UV absorption up to 400 nanometers" block 100 percent of UV light.

Make sure the lenses also block blue light. For that reason, brown to yellow lenses seem to work best. Many people with macular degeneration report that yellow lenses seem to increase the contrast in their visual field, which is very helpful when you have this disease.

Check for Distortion

Choose sunglasses with lenses that are completely free of distortion. This is especially important for people who already have symptoms of macular degeneration, since they may already have some distortion in their central field of view.

You can test for distortion in sunglass lenses by taking an Amsler Grid along when trying them on. Stare at the central dot and move the sunglass lenses around near the eye while staring at the dot. If any distortions appear, other than those that have been regularly charted, the lenses are not of high quality. In the absence of an Amsler Grid, use straight lines in the environment to test the lenses for distortion.

Design Matters

The design of sunglasses also affects how much they protect the eyes. Since light enters the eye from all directions, sunglasses should cover the entire eye. Several manufacturers make models that wrap around the sides of the eyes. Some even make models that cover the gaps formed above and below, between the frames and the eye socket. Several manufacturers make goggle-type sunglasses for active sports, which are useful for some people with macular degeneration.

Check Your Contact Lenses

Some people who wear contacts erroneously assume that they protect their eyes from UV light. Contact lenses that offer 100 percent protection from UV light must be labeled as such. If they are not, sunglasses are needed.

Use Caution in Special Lighting Conditions

Even the most protective sunglasses cannot adequately protect a person's eyes under special lighting conditions, such as the light from an arc welder, or staring at the sun during an eclipse. Wearing inadequate eye protection while looking at these light sources can cause a painful but temporary condition known as *photokeratitis*, an inflammation caused by intense light. Under extreme conditions, looking at these light sources can cause permanent loss of central vision. People who have macular degeneration should avoid these light sources.

People who have had cataract surgery should check with their surgeons to see if they used one of the newer, UV-absorbent implants. Older implants were not UV absorbent, so people who have those implants in their eyes will need to be extra careful about wearing a hat and sunglasses when outdoors.

Some Drugs May Intensify Sunlight

Certain drugs make the skin, and oftentimes the eyes, more sensitive to light. Macular degeneration patients taking such medications should be sure to discuss with their physician whether the drugs may cause photosensitivity of the eyes.

Commonly used drugs that do cause photosensitivity of the eyes include the tetracycline antibiotics, such as minocycline and doxycycline. The psoralen group of drugs, which includes Oxsoralen (methoxsalen), also cause photosensitivity. The psoralen drugs are used to treat psoriasis, skin pigments, and hair regrowth. Also, the class of drugs known as phenothiazines, used to treat psychiatric disorders and other medical problems, are known to cause photosensitivity of the eyes.

People who do take drugs that make the eyes sensitive to light should be sure to wear a hat and sunglasses at all times when outdoors, even if it is for a few minutes.

6

The Emotional Impact of Macular Degeneration

When you or a loved one is suddenly faced with a diagnosis of macular degeneration, you may feel emotionally devastated. It's easy to understand why. Our society is so visually oriented, and the loss of central vision can be frightening, especially if you face the prospect of losing some of your independence. Some individuals make the adjustment relatively easily; others sink into depression. Your reaction will probably depend, in part, on such things as the amount of support you have from friends and relatives. Whatever your situation, it is important to understand the psychological implications of having macular degeneration and to deal with them as effectively as you can.

Coping Emotionally

Having macular degeneration usually means more than simply the physical loss of sight, although that is difficult enough to deal with. As children and adults, we define much of our self-image by our sight. But, when your sight is compromised by macular degeneration, you may need to change your self-image from that of a sighted person to that of a visually handicapped person, which can be a difficult transition indeed.

If your visual loss is sudden, you may experience a period of shock, characterized by listlessness, inability to concentrate, depression, denial, anxiety, or a wide range of other physical symptoms.

It would be entirely normal for you to experience a mourning process for your lost vision, even though you may not realize it at the time. Some patients experience deep feelings of sadness and may spend blocks of time crying. Others may suddenly exhibit behaviors of dependency, even if they have been highly independent up to that point in their lives. Many patients become depressed or irritable or may show other symptoms following their initial reaction of shock.

On the pragmatic side, the perceived financial stresses of having macular degeneration sometimes increase a person's anxiety, as the individual anticipates expenses for specialized equipment, taxis, or house modifications. The fear of having costly and/or debilitating accidents, the inability to pay bills, or the apprehension of being unable to do common household tasks such as cooking may reinforce a person's fear of dependency.

However, when a person is allowed—even encouraged—to go through these emotional phases completely, the patient eventually accepts his or her visual limitations, seeks out helpful resources, and develops ways to adapt. Caregivers should encourage patients to talk about how they feel, even if it means repeated conversations covering similar emotional reactions.

It is important to recognize that two people with the same degree of vision loss may have very different psychological reactions and emotional needs. Much of a person's reaction depends on such factors as age of onset, the degree of vision loss, how quickly the disease progresses, one's ability to handle loss, lifestyle at the time of loss, and even individual biases toward visual handicaps or handicapped people.

Since macular degeneration typically affects older people, a person's reaction to the disease overlies any infirmities, feelings of isolation, or other emotional symptoms he/she may be experiencing due to aging. For example, a recent study found that older adults with vision loss have rates of depression between 31 percent and 40 percent, compared to 15 percent to 20 percent in the general population of the elderly.

Mary was 80 when she was first diagnosed with wet macular degeneration.

> *The diagnosis crushed me. I had been fiercely independent, and living alone, since my husband died some twenty years earlier. I felt despondent over my gradual loss of central vision. I'd seen too many of my friends lose vision and give up hope. I was scared. I began to live in seclusion. I neglected my appearance. I just didn't want to talk to anyone.*
>
> *Fortunately, my daughter had a long career in social services and recognized what was happening. She mobilized my friends and encouraged them to call or visit me just to listen to my fears. Through a macular degeneration support group in a nearby town, she found Agnes, a woman who had lived with macular degeneration for more than a decade and who maintained a positive attitude and an independent lifestyle. Agnes visited me and we hit it off immediately. It was the first time I had seen*

a person with macular degeneration who did not lose hope.

Within six weeks, I felt better. Agnes offered me advice every time I faced a barrier, and pretty soon I began to share my triumphs with my family and friends. Now I realize how Agnes helped reignite my positive attitude toward life. Of course I'd rather not have macular degeneration, but overall I feel as if I've adjusted well to it.

Despite the negative reactions to macular degeneration, many people experience significant emotional and spiritual growth as an outgrowth of dealing with the disease. If you commit to making the best of the disease, you will soon realize that hope, humor, patience, and a positive attitude make a huge difference in living an independent lifestyle.

Tips for Coping

- Talk about emotions. Share feelings of loneliness or dependency.
- Use humor to reduce stress. It is inevitable that macular degeneration will cause embarrassing situations to occur. For example, your first attempts at eating in a formal setting may be awkward. Humor goes a long way in defusing tension and anxiety.
- Keep up spiritual practices or consider renewing them. Faith helps people facing a disease such as macular degeneration.
- Keep a positive attitude. Every situation is a challenge with hidden opportunities for personal growth. Look for those opportunities. Carve out time for personal pursuits.

- Ask for help. You are providing an opportunity for others to feel good about helping.
- Meet other people with low vision. Share your feelings, self-doubts, and difficult challenges with them. Ask for advice on how they handle specific challenges.
- Be patient. Learning to cope with macular degeneration takes time and energy, but eventually nearly all patients reach a comfortable balance with the disease.
- Learn as much as possible about macular degeneration, how to deal with the challenges it presents, and new treatments on the horizon. Discuss any questions with a retinal specialist.
- Get regular exercise, but consult with a physician first.

Bill S., a retired executive, was 70 when he was diagnosed with macular degeneration.

I'll never forget the day I was diagnosed with macular degeneration. I was upset but not really devastated by the diagnosis. I guess my take-charge attitude took over. On my next visit to my doctor, I had a list of questions that carried over to a second sheet of paper.

I learned I had a complex form of macular degeneration. There were a lot of treatments, which were annoying because they took up time. I'd rather have used the time for other things, like the macular degeneration support group I joined. I put together a comedy night for them every month, where people with macular degeneration and our families tell jokes, raise money to help find cures for the disease and, most of all, enjoy ourselves.

Tips for Family, Friends, and Caregivers

The attitude of family, friends, and caregivers can affect the state of mind of a person with macular degeneration and his/her adjustment to the disease. It's important to understand that those with macular degeneration can see peripherally. However, they have difficulty with central vision, which is necessary for reading and other tasks that require fine vision, including recognizing faces. Unless complications arise, their visual loss is confined to their central vision. That is why it's helpful for caregivers to ask patients with macular degeneration what degree of visual loss they have, so care can be planned accordingly.

- Use whatever adaptive mechanisms are available to keep the patient functioning as independently as possible.

- Encourage the patient to express feelings and allow time for the grieving process to resolve itself. Even with patients who have long ago adjusted to their macular degeneration, new demands on their lifestyle can trigger frustration, angry reactions, or temporary depression. Allow time for the patient to work through each of these episodes.

- If caregivers feel that a patient's reaction is beyond normal bounds, or is lasting too long, they should encourage the patient to seek professional counseling or to join one of the many support groups that are available (see appendix).

- Macular degeneration by its very nature is stress-producing, as the patient must constantly adapt to challenging situations. Stress makes adjustments to living with macular degeneration more difficult and increases one's vulnerability to illness. Encourage the patient to incorporate stress-relieving strategies into his/her daily routine. Stress-reducing activities include meditation, tai chi, walking or other exercise, deep breathing, frequent discussions to allow the patient to express feelings, healthy eating, humor, and a good support network.

- Avoid the desire to overprotect a person with macular degeneration. Encourage the person to be self-reliant and as independent as the disability allows. Allow the person to help with chores or contribute in other ways to the maintenance of the household.

- Speak in a normal tone of voice. Macular degeneration does not affect hearing.

- When entering or leaving a visually impaired person's space, announce your arrival and departure. Similarly, tell the person when you are about to do something within his/her personal space. If others are in the room when the patient enters, be sure to introduce them.

- Be direct when asking to help. When offering walking assistance, offer your arm. Do not just grab a patient's arm. Then walk at a normal pace, hesitating before stairs or other obstacles. It is a good idea to describe in advance for the person the new areas you are entering.

- Don't hesitate to describe surroundings, since at one point the person with macular degeneration was normally sighted and usually appreciates such cues.

- Be mindful of helpful gifts on special occasions. Consider gifts of concert tickets, a talking clock, or a book on tape.

- Don't avoid words like see ("It was nice to *see* you") or *look* ("Wow, *look* at that!"). Just be sure to describe the interesting items in view.

- People with macular degeneration should be encouraged to read and use their eyes as much as possible. With consistent use, visual acuity may actually increase.
- Encourage the patient to begin new hobbies, such as gardening, playing a musical instrument, or learning how to use a computer.
- When writing notes to a person with macular degeneration, print using a black felt-tipped marker on bright white paper.
- Help boost the patient's self-esteem by recognizing his/her efforts and praising each new accomplishment.

Reaching Out to the Community

According to one national survey, only one in five patients knows that visual rehabilitation services are available, and only 2 percent actually use those services. If you have macular degeneration, consider taking advantage of the many rehabilitation services that are available (see appendix). These programs help teach patients how to restructure their daily activities to successfully cope with low vision and maintain as high a degree of independence as possible.

- One of the most effective and low-cost aids is a support person or group of people with macular degeneration. Patients report that such meetings offer an emotional boost and practical advice for coping with the challenges of daily activities. Exchange telephone numbers and E-mail addresses so that you can reach out to one another between meetings.
- Beyond support groups, most medium and large communities offer a wide range of services to people dealing with macular degeneration. The federal

government offers a program known as "Independent Living Services for Older Individuals Who Are Blind." Actually, the title of the program is a misnomer, since it also offers services to people over the age of 55 who are not totally blind. The program is run by individual states, so check with state offices to determine eligibility and services offered.

- Rehabilitation centers offer people with macular degeneration an opportunity to learn new ways to handle daily activities such as cooking, computing, and personal care. The National Rehabilitation Information Center (see appendix) offers a list of centers in every region of the country.

- State and county governments are the principal conduits for information and services related to visual impairments. Increasingly, the list of available services can be determined by both telephone and Web site. Typical places to search in the telephone directory are under Department of Aging, Administration on Aging, Department of Rehabilitation, and Department of Social and Health Services. Most states offer rehabilitation programs designed to encourage and maintain independent living.

- Finally, a number of nonprofit groups offer services through their local chapters. Organizations such as the American Foundation for the Blind, the American Council for the Blind, and the National Association for the Visually Handicapped all offer a wealth of information and programs for people with visual handicaps. Some also offer scholarships to visually impaired people for postsecondary education or serve as conduits for government scholarships.

7

Choosing an Eye Care Team

The best way to reduce your risk of vision loss due to macular degeneration is to create a well-functioning eye care team. Older patients may feel uncomfortable consciously choosing health-care providers. But, only by employing the strengths of each team member can you be certain that the best effort is being made to protect your vision. In many cases, putting the eye care team together requires that you, a friend, or a family member serve as quarterback. Some practices have already assembled teams to better serve the medical needs of their patients. Those needs are not limited to surgery or medications. They include empathetic listening, developing a prevention program when possible, effective monitoring of telltale signs of potential vision loss, and good communication with the eye care team members.

Sometimes patients delay contacting a physician because of discomfort with how they were treated by a former physician or support staff. In other cases, a physician may not take the time to develop and explain how to vigilantly conduct an ongoing monitoring program. These situations can and do result in further damage to the retina and possible further loss of sight.

Types of Eye Doctors

To optimize your eye care team, it is important to understand the expertise and role of each of its members. Eye doctors who can help with macular degeneration are optometrists, general ophthalmologists, and retinal specialists.

Optometrists

Optometrists are licensed to perform certain components of general eye care. Optometrists attend a school of optometry for four years after graduating from college. In addition, some optometrists spend an additional year of training as a resident. After graduating, they specialize in general eye exams and prescribing eyeglass lenses and contact lenses. In most states, optometrists can also prescribe eyedrops and certain oral medicines. However, optometrists are not licensed to perform laser treatments or surgery in most states.

General Ophthalmologists

Ophthalmologists are licensed medical doctors. They are able to perform eye exams, prescribe eyeglasses and contact lenses, and prescribe eyedrops as well as all other medicines. Ophthalmologists undergo a minimum of four years of additional training after medical school. The first year is usually spent as an intern in general surgery or internal medicine, followed by a three- or four-year ophthalmology residency. Ophthalmologists can also perform eye surgery, but the specific types of surgery each ophthalmologist performs depend upon his or her specialty.

Some ophthalmologists specialize in cataract surgery, others in corneal surgery such as laser refractive surgery (LASIK). Still others specialize in surgery of the retina. Each subspecialty of ophthalmology, including treatment of the retina, is very demanding and requires significant experience and expertise in order to be optimally effective.

Retinal Specialists

Retinal specialists are highly trained in the diagnosis, management, and treatment of retinal problems such as macular degeneration, retinal detachment, diabetic retinopathy, and macular holes; retinopathy refers to abnormal function of the retinal blood vessels due to diabetes, and macular holes refer to holes that may develop in the center of the macula. Retinal specialists typically undergo two additional years of extensive training after getting their ophthalmology certificate. This extra training is called a *fellowship*. This is a very complex and demanding subspecialty and typically occupies all the time of ophthalmologists who specialize in treating the retina.

Beside the patient, the retinal specialist is the most important member of the macular degeneration management team. A good retinal specialist should assist you in developing a manageable prevention program based upon solid scientific information that is explained in a way that you can readily understand. That means the retinal specialist should also be a good listener.

The retinal specialist should advise you on an individualized and workable early detection and monitoring program, and should be able to provide a host of standard and cutting-edge treatments that can be individualized to your needs and extent of macular degeneration. The specialist should also explain various treatment options and have the courage to make recommendations with your best interests at heart, even if you may not initially agree with those recommendations.

How to Select an Eye Doctor

Many people feel uncomfortable with the notion of interviewing and selecting an eye doctor. Instead, they act by default. They simply go to the first doctor recommended and try to "make the best of it."

Communication between you and your doctor should be comfortable and effective. Interviewing a physician does not have to be the daunting task that many people imagine it to be. It is simply a way for you and your physician to get to know one another and see if you can work together to actively and effectively manage your illness. Patients who go into the process with a positive attitude have a much better outcome. Generally, it is best to conduct the interview after the doctor has had a chance to take a medical history and examine your eyes. Then the doctor can respond to your questions more specifically.

Selecting a physician ideally involves three distinct phases: observing, questioning, and evaluating. For you to obtain the best possible fit with a doctor, it is important to cover as many of the following questions as possible at some time during the selection process. It often helps to have a friend or family member along to be sure that the most critical questions are answered.

Observe the Staff

- Is the staff attentive to my needs and compassionate when discussing my medical issues?
- Is the staff respectful of my time and medical needs?
- Is the staff knowledgeable? Ask questions about what you have learned from this book regarding macular degeneration and its treatments.

- Does the staff believe in their doctors? Strange as it may seem, just ask them point-blank.

Observe the Office

- Is the waiting room comfortable?
- Is the waiting room handicapped accessible?
- Is pertinent, up-to-date information available in the waiting room? Is the material generic and supplied by various professional societies, or did the practice take the trouble to develop its own material?
- How long must I wait to see the doctor? Given the fact that a patient may need to have his/her eyes dilated, it may take thirty to forty-five minutes. Any longer is generally excessive unless there is an extreme, unexpected emergency. In that case, the staff owes the patient regular updates without the patient having to ask.

Observe the Doctor

- Is the doctor attentive and compassionate?
- Does the doctor give me his/her full attention?
- Do I feel comfortable talking with the doctor?
- Does the doctor and the staff make careful notes about my condition?
- Does the doctor offer realistic hope?

Questions to Ask the Doctor

- How many patients with macular degeneration do you see per week?
- How many years have you been seeing patients with macular degeneration?
- What are my options for prevention of vision loss?

- What are my options and risks for treatment with dry macular degeneration?
- What are my options and risks for treatment with wet macular degeneration?
- How do you track your results of treatment?
- What are your results? Are they different for each treatment type?
- May I have a copy of your résumé (known as a CV, for curriculum vitae)?
- How do you view your role in the care or prevention of my macular degeneration?
- Will you work closely with my optometrist, primary care physician, and general ophthalmologist to come up with an effective treatment and management plan?
- How active are you in training other physicians?
- Do you conduct research involving cutting-edge treatments? Have you published the results of that research? May I have a copy of some of those articles?
- What type of continuing medical education have you taken recently?
- May I have a few recent patient references to contact?

Interview Other Patients and Eye Care Providers

Interviewing references is often *the* most important thing a person can do to increase the odds that the physician will be the right choice. Ask the doctor for references from other patients and from other eye care providers. Call everyone on the list. When interviewing other patients, consider asking:

- How long have you been in the care of the doctor?

- What do you consider to be his/her major strengths? How do those strengths show up in his/her care for you?
- What do you consider to be his/her major weaknesses? How do those weaknesses show up in your treatment?
- Does the doctor allow adequate time to answer all your questions? Does he/she encourage you to call between visits with questions you may have? Does he/she respond to questions by E-mail?
- Are you satisfied with your treatment? Does the doctor explain all options available to you? Does he/she encourage you to discuss other treatment options you may have heard about? Has he/she been candid and realistic about your prognosis?
- When interviewing other eye care specialists as references, consider asking:
  - Why do you recommend this person so highly?
  - Have other of your patients seen this doctor? What were the results?
  - Is this the physician you would refer yourself or your family members to for similar medical problems?

Evaluate

With the basic observations and interviews now over, evaluate the physicians to determine which one is best for your specific situation and needs. It is often helpful to discuss your perceptions with one or more family members or with a trusted friend. This is also a good time for you to call the doctor's office to clarify answers to some of the questions. Once you choose a physician, schedule a follow-up appointment immediately.

Office Visits: Hints for Better Communication

Once you have selected an eye care team, it is important to make sure that subsequent visits achieve their objectives. Before each visit, ask yourself:

- Why am I seeing the doctor? Am I here for a routine eye exam, a specific concern, or to talk about a lifestyle change?
- What do I want to gain from this visit?
- What lifestyle changes (diet, exercise, quitting smoking, etc.) can the doctor suggest to improve my health?

Keep a running list and note any health problems that are secondary to the major reason for your visit. If any new health problems arise, tell the doctor at the start that you have other areas of concern that may or may not be relevant to the primary reason for the visit.

Patients who ask questions of their doctor have much higher rates of compliance with subsequent appointments and measurably better health outcomes. In other words, better communication translates into better health. This principle is also important when talking with a physician's assistant, nurse, or technician. If you have questions, ask them.

It also helps if a patient knows what to expect from a doctor's visit. Every doctor must play detective, teasing out the critical symptoms from irrelevant information until a reasonable diagnosis can be made. To get to a good diagnosis, doctors typically take a brief history and a summary of the complaint, conduct physical exam, then have a consultation after the exam. The physician should tell the patient what to expect during the visit, what they are doing, and what will happen next.

The initial visit is a good time to discuss a particular medication, test, or procedure that you have heard of and that you think may be helpful.

However, it is up to you to make sure that your needs are being addressed. Be clear in your own mind why you have scheduled the visit. Was it only for blurry vision, or are there other vision issues of concern? Sometimes second or third medical problems can be as troublesome as the one that originally brought you to the doctor.

Communication Is the Key

It may be reassuring to know that most doctors today give a great deal of thought to promoting open communication with their patients. The issue of patients being able to make informed treatment decisions based on sound medical advice is an important principle of medical ethics. The doctor should be willing to actively listen to your questions. If you do not feel that this is happening, say so. If the problem continues, consider getting another doctor. Patients who arrive with questions and are ready to take notes are better prepared for their visit, leave with the information they wanted, and are better in following up on the treatment plan.

Agree on a Point of Contact

Before leaving the office after the initial visit, have a clear agreement with the physician as to whom to contact to discuss visual changes. Does the doctor wish to be contacted directly? If so, what times are best? How long should you wait for a reply before calling again? Does the doctor instead prefer that a knowledgeable nurse or technician take the information? Many practices do this and share the information with the supervising doctor several times a day. Then the nurse or technician will call the patient back with advice. In certain instances, the doctor may call back to get more information.

Give Your Doctor Feedback

Finally, if you are not happy with how a physician handles your medical care, or if you feel mistreated by the receptionist, technicians, billing manager, or anyone else in the practice, let your physician know. You should always feel as if you and your doctors are a team whose mission it is to treat and prevent macular degeneration under the best conditions possible.

8

Treatments for Macular Degeneration

Great strides have been made in the treatment of wet macular degeneration in recent years, although treatments for dry macular degeneration are just beginning to be developed. The reason? Wet macular degeneration has a more rapid progression, typically over a period of weeks or months. It is easier to develop treatments for a condition that develops rapidly because a physician can immediately see if his/her efforts work. Dry macular degeneration usually progresses slowly, over a period of many years. Therefore, results of experimental treatments are not known for years, making it more difficult to develop treatments for the dry type.

Treating Dry Macular Degeneration

Many patients are frustrated by the lack of treatment for dry macular degeneration. They may feel their condition is a ticking time bomb and there is no way to defuse it. Dry macular degeneration may not turn into the wet form for many years, and if it does, health-care professionals do not yet have any way to predict when it will appear. Meantime, one's risk can be reduced.

Reducing Risk

Despite the current lack of effective treatments, a person can reduce the risk or delay the progression of dry macular degeneration. These prevention practices are detailed in chapter 5 and consist of a proper diet, regular exercise, use of good quality sunglasses, controlling high cholesterol and blood pressure, consuming alcohol in moderation, and quitting smoking.

Early Detection Is Key

Aside from prevention efforts, early detection is important to reducing one's risk of vision loss. Be diligent about daily eye self-examinations and regular visits to an eye care professional. Any changes in vision whatsoever may signal the transformation of dry into the more serious and damaging wet macular degeneration. Therefore, any changes in vision should be reported *immediately* to an eye care professional. A delay of even a few weeks can mean irreversible damage to central vision.

Treating Wet Macular Degeneration

Current treatment for wet macular degeneration involves either reducing the leakage of the abnormal blood vessels under the retina or moving the central portion of the retina, the macula, away from the leaking blood vessels.

Photodynamic Treatment

This form of treatment is used in cases in which 50 percent of the leakage is the "classic" or most rapid form. The treatment involves injecting a drug into the body. When the drug reaches the eye, a special laser activates the drug to control the leaking blood vessels. In the past, the surgical laser used had a high-energy, continuous beam of light. That light caused heat to build just under the retina. Unfortunately, that heat also damaged the retina.

A newer technique, photodynamic treatment avoids the overheating problem. This treatment uses a dye that is injected into the blood through a vein; the dye accumulates in the abnormal, leaking blood vessels under the retina. *Visudyne* is the name of the first of these dyes to prove its effectiveness in clinical trials, and others are expected to become available soon. Once activated, chemicals in the dye close the leaking blood vessels. A laser delivers the colored light necessary to activate the dye. This laser is of sufficiently low intensity that it does not cause any significant heat damage by itself. For this reason it is often called a "cold" laser.

Although photodynamic treatment causes less damage to the retina than older laser treatments, some damage may still occur. That damage is probably responsible for the finding that photodynamic treatment as currently used seldom improves vision. Retinal specialists are hopeful that with continued development of photodynamic treatments, damage to the retina can be further reduced. This might require new dyes or improved lasers, both of which are being researched.

How the Treatment Is Performed

The surgeon first maps the area of leakage by using special dyes that are injected into the bloodstream and travel to the eye. The area is photographed and the laser is set up to deliver the proper wavelength of light. The surgeon also determines the correct dose of photodynamic dye that is needed. The dye is then injected slowly, over the course of several minutes, through a vein in the patient's arm.

After an additional several minutes to allow the dye to concentrate in the leaking blood vessels of the eye, the low-intensity laser is focused on them by using a contact lens temporarily placed on the eye. The contact lens is removed as soon as the treatment is completed. The laser is focused on the leaking blood vessels for a little more than a minute in order to sufficiently activate the dye. While the treatment itself only takes several minutes, considerable time is necessary to properly plan the treatment, so the patient may actually spend an hour or more undergoing this procedure.

The laser procedure is performed at a *biomicroscope station,* which consists of a special stand where the patient rests his/her chin and forehead, and a specially designed microscope that allows the surgeon to see the retina. The patient's vision in the treated eye may seem dark for a few hours after treatment because the light-sensing cells have been saturated with light from the procedure. The darkness will then usually disappear.

Other than a needle stick in the arm to put in the dye, there is usually no pain or discomfort during the treatment, although occasionally some patients report temporary back pain. After treatment, patients are usually advised to protect themselves from direct sunlight and to wear sunglasses for several days.

Treatment Outcomes

Photodynamic treatment typically slows the rate of vision loss. It usually takes five to six treatments over the course of one to two years to slow the progression of macular degeneration.

It is important for patients to be aware that photodynamic treatment as it is currently performed very rarely improves vision. It is also rare to totally stop vision loss until about eighteen to twenty-four months after treatment is begun.

As photodynamic treatment is refined, physicians hope that some visual improvement will be achieved using it or by combining it with other techniques. Fortunately, there are other techniques that can improve vision in certain individuals with wet macular degeneration.

Transpupillary Thermotherapy

Transpupillary thermotherapy (*TTT*) involves the use of long-wavelength *infrared light* to reduce blood vessel leakage. Infrared light, which cannot be seen by humans, penetrates more deeply into human tissue than does visible light. When focused on leaking blood vessels under the retina, infrared light tends to cause a small temperature elevation in those blood vessels. That rise in temperature tends to close some of the leaking blood vessels, with minimal damage to the retina. However, there is a trade-off. Because of the more modest temperature elevation, the ability to totally stop the leakage and seal the blood vessels may be reduced.

How the Treatment Is Performed

The preparation for TTT is much like that for photodynamic treatment. Angiograms are taken to determine the characteristics of the leaking blood vessels under the retina. The blood vessels that respond best to TTT are those that have mostly occult, or the least rapid form of leakage. However, investigations are underway to determine the role TTT may have in treating other leaking blood vessels.

The area of leakage is then mapped and the laser adjusted to deliver the proper dose of light. A contact lens is then temporarily placed on the eye to focus the beam, and the infrared laser is applied.

Treatment is not painful. The patient's vision in the treated eye may seem dark for a few hours after treatment. The darkness will then usually go away. The treatment itself takes only 20 to 30 minutes, although an hour or more may be necessary to properly plan the treatment.

Treatment Outcomes

TTT may slow the rate of vision loss. This treatment usually does not result in significant improvement of vision, although in some cases it can. Occasionally, TTT can cause some decline in vision. In the occasional cases where vision improves after TTT, the improvement often progresses slowly over several months.

Feeder Vessel Treatment

The idea behind *feeder vessel treatment* is to close the blood vessel that feeds the leaking area, just as you might stop the flow of nutrients to a leaf by pinching off the stem. Feeder vessel treatment was significantly advanced through the development of a very special dye (ICG) and high-speed, computer-aided photography. The technology is called *high-speed ICG angiography*. This tool allows your doctor to evaluate the blood vessel leakage and other changes occurring in wet macular degeneration vastly better than ever before. This newer technology represents a great breakthrough for people suffering from wet macular degeneration.

Due to the microscopic size of these feeder vessels, highly focused, pinpoint lasers must be used. These lasers allow retinal surgeons to focus the laser energy on the deeper areas where the feeder vessels are found. This reduces the potential damage to the retina dramatically and enhances the effectiveness of the treatment.

If new feeder vessels develop or previous feeder vessels reopen, the use of these pinpoint lasers makes repeat treatment also relatively low risk. Feeder vessel treatment targets the problem at a very basic level and tends to create a healthier blood flow for the eye. In effect, feeder vessel treatment fine-tunes the blood supply to the eye.

How the Treatment Is Performed

The network of blood vessels under the retina is carefully mapped using two specialized dyes, high-speed, high-resolution digital cameras, and high-speed computers. The feeder vessels are usually visible for only a second or two. Although the treatment of feeder vessels has been carried out for more than thirty years, the technology making it possible to more accurately detect and map them in macular degeneration has only been available within the past few years. Prior to this, feeder vessels could be detected in only a small fraction of people with wet macular degeneration. With this new technology, feeder vessels can be detected in more than 80 percent of eyes with wet macular degeneration.

To get the right pictures, a tiny needle is placed in a vein in the patient's arm to deliver the dye. Only a very tiny amount of each dye is currently required due to the greater sensitivity of the new cameras. In fact, the amount of dye required has been reduced fourfold over the past few years as camera sensitivity has improved. These tiny amounts of dye are generally very well tolerated and very safe.

The process of scanning the retina as the dye travels through the blood vessels takes only about twenty or thirty minutes. However, considerable time is often required to analyze and interpret the results. In uncomplicated cases the analysis can be done in less than an hour, but in more complex cases it may take several hours.

Using high-speed computers, the retinal surgeon analyzes the microscopic flow of blood supplying the retina. The feeder vessel or vessels are carefully mapped. Using this map, the surgeon treats them with the pinpoint laser, reducing the amount of laser energy used to less than one thousandth of that which was previously required.

As in other treatments, the laser procedure is performed at a biomicroscope station. The patient's vision in the treated eye will seem dark for a few hours after treatment. The darkness will almost always completely go away. The laser treatment itself may take 15 to 20 minutes. However, to properly plan the treatment the physician may require several hours and may even need to schedule the treatment the following day.

Multiple treatments over the course of a few weeks are sometimes needed, depending upon the number and size of the feeder vessels identified. Consequently, earlier treatment is desirable since feeder vessels enlarge and multiply with time, yet another reason to detect macular degeneration as early as possible.

> *When I was diagnosed with wet macular degeneration, I immediately researched my options and found a surgeon who was familiar with the feeder vessel procedure. It was a good thing, because shortly after I had an episode of bleeding under the retina which compromised my sight. I thank God that I got to my surgeon in time. He did the surgery and actually improved my sight!*
>
> —Fred C.

Treatment Outcomes

The goal of feeder vessel treatment is to stabilize or even improve vision. Success is often dependent upon the duration of leakage prior to treatment. The longer that blood and fluid have been present under the retina, the more scarring and deterioration of the retina may have occurred.

Success also depends on the size, complexity, and number of feeder vessels. The longer that the abnormal vessels are present, the larger and more complex they become. As a consequence, the complexity of treatment increases the longer the leakage is present. Therefore, early treatment is beneficial in order to achieve best results. In addition, if the blood and fluid under the retina are very thick, it becomes more difficult to detect the feeder vessels and adequately treat them with the laser.

Many of these limitations can be at least partially overcome with repeated treatments. Fortunately, since both the area and the intensity of the laser treatment is so small, multiple treatments are well tolerated. In a minority of cases, improvement of vision can occur within hours or days. These are often cases where the fluid was present only for a few days or weeks and the fluid was not thickened or bloody. More commonly, vision improves gradually over the course of several weeks to several months, with some patients taking as long as two years to notice improvements. During this time, several treatment sessions may be required.

As vision improves, people often notice a decrease in distortion or increase in color perception. Sometimes the central dark spot begins to diminish, becoming less dark—often gray—so that some images can be seen through it. Sometimes the central black area breaks up so the patient begins to see through what appear to be holes in it.

Although vision improvement can occur, and in some cases can be substantial, vision is usually not going to return to the near-perfect level that was experienced prior to the leakage. It is important to remember that without treatment most forms of wet macular degeneration cause continued deterioration of central vision over one to several years. In some cases where the treatment is not successful in reducing leakage, continued vision loss may occur.

Intravitreal Bubble to Displace Blood Under the Retina

This procedure uses a gas or air bubble placed within the eye to apply pressure to the retina and thereby push blood out from under the macula. This treatment is used predominantly in cases where there is so much blood and/or thickened fluid under the retina that it blocks the ability to see and treat the leaking blood vessels with any other treatments. Once the blockage is removed, other treatments can then be used to reduce or stop further leakage.

In a large number of circumstances over the past thirty years, bubbles have been injected into the vitreous cavity of the eye—the central portion of the eye filled with a clear, jelly-like fluid. The bubbles are used to apply gentle internal pressure to push a detached retina back into place, to push down the elevated edges of a macular hole or retinal tear, and to stop bleeding.

How the Treatment Is Performed

A bubble of gas or air is placed into the vitreous cavity of the eye with a very thin needle. The bubble floats up to the highest point, where it pushes upwards with gentle pressure. Depending upon the type and mixture of gases, the bubble remains within the eye for days to weeks. The amount of problematic blood present in the eye often influences the time the bubble is designed to stay before it is absorbed by the eye.

In order for the bubble to be positioned to push the blood away from the center of the retina, the patient must keep his or her head in a face-down position. It is usually recommended that patients keep their heads in a face-down position for 90 percent of the day for three to fourteen days. This allows about two and a half hours during the course of the day to keep one's head up for washing, eating, and other activities. Obviously this is not a pleasant situation, but most patients willingly do it to improve their sight.

Some surgeons will inject the gas or air bubble into the vitreous cavity of the eye in their office, under local anesthesia. This is a procedure with minimal pain and discomfort. Some surgeons feel that injecting a drug that helps dissolve clots at the same time as the bubble is introduced is helpful, but others feel that the clot-dissolving drug has no benefit.

Some surgeons feel that their results are better and the potential for complications is reduced if the procedure is performed in the operating room where any pain can be better managed and some of the vitreous gel can be removed when the bubble is placed in the vitreous cavity. They believe that removing the vitreous gel makes placement of the bubble safer. It also reduces the chances of the vitreous pulling on the delicate retina, which might cause repeat bleeding. Furthermore, a larger bubble can be placed in the eye if a portion of the vitreous gel is removed. Removal of the vitreous gel also reduces the possibility of bothersome "floaters," tiny dots that sometimes appear in the patient's field of vision after the procedure. The vitreous is frequently removed today, and its removal causes few, if any, problems.

After the procedure, however it is performed, the eye will feel a bit irritated for a few days. It will also appear a little red with perhaps a slight amount of blood drainage. The bubble blocks vision for a few days to a few weeks, depending on the duration of action of the bubble. The body reabsorbs the bubble normally. There is never a case where the bubble of gas or air fails to be reabsorbed.

Vision will usually gradually improve over the ensuing few weeks to months. During that time, angiography will be performed and additional treatment to stop any re-bleeding will likely be undertaken. In some cases, leakage from the abnormal blood vessels under the retina stops after the bubble presses on the blood vessels for a while. In these cases, additional treatment might not be required.

Placement of a bubble in the vitreous cavity can cause cataracts to develop. This complication can be reduced somewhat by adhering to the face-down position recommended by the surgeon. A bubble can also result in a retinal tear and detachment. These can be repaired successfully in the vast majority of cases, but their occurrence would require further surgery.

Treatment Outcomes

Although some improvement of vision can be achieved, the main benefit of treatment is to allow the use of other treatments to directly reduce blood vessel leakage.

Central Vision-Sparing Direct Laser Treatment

The *central vision-sparing direct laser treatment* is intended to stop leaking blood vessels that do not involve the most visually sensitive area of the central macula, the fovea. It is rarely performed today due to the availability of other surgical procedures.

How the Treatment Is Performed

The network of blood vessels under the retina is carefully mapped using a specialized dye, computerized cameras, and computers. The dye clearly shows the area of leaking blood vessels. The retinal specialist then uses this information to apply laser treatment to the entire area of leaking blood vessels.

The process takes only about twenty or thirty minutes, although considerable time is required to analyze and interpret the results.

As in other treatments, the laser procedure is performed at a biomicroscope station, which serves to hold the patient's head very still. The patient's vision in the treated eye will seem dark for a few hours after treatment. However, the darkness will usually diminish significantly over the next few days.

Treatment Outcomes

Central vision-sparing direct laser treatment usually can slow the progression of visual loss. In certain cases vision can be stabilized or even improved. Central vision-sparing direct laser treatment is limited by the fact that fewer than five percent of patients with wet macular degeneration have leaking blood vessels not involving the fovea or center of the macula. New leakage subsequently reoccurs in 50 to 65 percent of cases within three years of treatment. The new leakage is almost always under the fovea, making further treatment using this procedure impossible. The main risk to the patient is that laser treatment may damage some of the fovea, since treatment often must be applied very close to it.

Treatment to Relocate the Macula

Macular Translocation

As its name implies, *macular translocation* is a surgical procedure that moves the center of the macula away from the leaking blood vessels. Once this is accomplished, the leaking blood vessels are treated with a direct, high-energy laser. The portions of the more peripheral retina that are damaged by the laser treatment do not interfere significantly with central vision.

How the Treatment Is Performed

Macular translocation is performed as an outpatient procedure in an operating room. Local anesthesia and sedation are generally required. A variety of surgical techniques are currently being used. They all require detachment of a major portion of the retina and then reattachment of the retina after it is shifted or rotated to move the center of the macula away from the area of leakage. Once this is done, an intravitreal bubble is introduced to keep the retina in place with gentle pressure.

After surgery the patient usually has to position his/her head in a face-down position for a few days to a couple of weeks. The exact positioning of the head is dependent upon the surgical technique used and the position of the leaking blood vessels.

Treatment Outcomes

If the macula can be moved enough to be positioned on healthy, non-leaking blood vessels and if the retina has not already suffered some damage from leakage and scarring, vision may improve.

Due to shifting of the retina, double vision can be a problem in some patients. Sometimes patients can adapt to the double vision. In other cases, prisms built into a patient's glasses may help. Otherwise, surgical modification of the muscles surrounding the eye that control eye position and movement can reduce or eliminate double vision. Some surgeons modify these muscles at the time of macular translocation.

Cataract formation frequently occurs within months to years following macular translocation. Major hemorrhage within the eye can also occur during surgery. This is relatively uncommon but can cause severe loss of vision if the blood cannot be removed.

Since retinal detachment is a part of macular translocation surgery, a significant complication is re-detachment of the retina within weeks to months following surgery.

Lastly, in some cases the area of abnormal, leaking blood vessels grows and spreads even after successful treatment. Unfortunately, this growth is almost always directed toward the central area of the macula. In this situation all the initial problems to the retina caused by leakage can return. However, in cases where these complications do not occur or can be successfully managed, useful vision can often be restored.

Future Treatments

Although strides have been made in treating macular degeneration, the future holds promise for more effective treatments for both the dry and wet forms of the disease. Some of the treatment research involves drugs to control blood vessel growth and leakage as well as drugs to help the retina heal and grow new cells. Other future treatments might include radiation therapy to stop bleeding, replacement of retinal cells, the use of stem cells to generate new retinal cells, filtering potentially harmful substances from the blood, and even attempts to implant a retinal microchip.

9

Making the Home Eye-Friendly

I n our visually oriented society, having a visual disability as significant as macular degeneration is difficult for patients and their families. However, despite the emotional issues and physical limitations that macular degeneration imposes, there is much a person can do to cope with macular degeneration and even thrive.

Coping with macular degeneration begins in the home. People spend a lifetime making their homes as comfortable as possible. Then, in a period of months, macular degeneration can make the home unsafe, full of obstacles and frustrations that threaten their safety, independence, and feelings of self-worth. However, people with macular degeneration can continue to live independently in their own homes if they make them more *eye-friendly*.

Many of the specialty items suggested in this chapter, such as telephones with extra-large numbers, can be ordered through the catalog retailers listed in the appendix.

Lighting

The first step to making a home comfortable and safe is to make sure that lighting is optimal. That means lots of light of the appropriate type.

- Reduce glare. Use halogen bulbs wherever possible, since they produce less glare than regular incandescent or fluorescent bulbs. Lamp shades also reduce glare. Window coverings such as curtains, shades, blinds, or shutters should be used to reduce glare during the brightest times of the day.

- When reading, especially, use bright, focused halogen lights. Position these lights in key locations throughout the house: next to favorite reading chairs, at the bedside, near telephones, near the pantry, on desks, over the kitchen table, near the stove for reading recipes, and at the inside entranceway to sign for packages. A bright, focused light should be used on the exterior entranceway so that guests are easily recognized.

- Use night-lights in any rooms a person with macular degeneration will typically walk through at night. This is better than turning on bright lights at night, since people with macular degeneration adjust more slowly to changes in light.

- Once the light for a room is well balanced, hook that setting up to a single control unit so that lighting level can be achieved with the flick of one switch. Simple lighting control units are available at major hardware stores, or an electrician can configure an entire room or home system.

- Make it a habit to always carry a flashlight. Small flashlights are available in hardware stores or through catalogs. Keep plenty of fresh batteries on hand.

- Increasing the contrast between light and dark objects helps enormously. Wherever possible, place dark furniture in front of light walls, or a light-colored lamp next to a dark chair.

- When refurbishing lighting, do not forget to illuminate hallways, closets, stairs, pantries, attic, and basement. These areas are sources of frustration and even danger for people with macular degeneration.

- When decorating, avoid the use of intricate patterns. They can make it difficult to judge distance.

Bathroom and Personal Hygiene

Consistency and routine are important coping mechanisms for dealing with macular degeneration, especially when it comes to personal hygiene.

- Keep everything on the bathroom counter in the same place. Every time an item is used, be sure to return it to the same spot. Buy toiletries in different-shaped containers, or immediately transfer the contents to specifically earmarked dispensers.

- Use a dark-colored toothbrush with white toothpaste to increase contrast. Keeping one finger along the side of the brush helps guide the toothpaste. Some patients simply squeeze the toothpaste directly into their mouths.

- Learn to use and trust other senses, such as touch and smell, when checking whether the correct item is about to be used.

- Attach a magnifying mirror to the wall near the vanity so that it will not be misplaced or accidentally knocked onto the floor. Better yet, install a magnifying mirror with a bright light source integrated into one unit. These units are available from large hardware suppliers, electricians, and catalogs.

- If the bathroom has light-colored walls, sinks, and fixtures, use darker-colored soaps, tissues, and toilet paper to increase contrast.

- Keep wardrobes in neutral colors so outfits will match. Section wardrobes by color for easier selection. Attach large labels to hangers dedicated to specific pieces of clothing. Then mix and match according to that labeling scheme. For example, label the hangers holding all tops with large letters. Then label matching pants with both the letter of the top that it matches, plus a number. Some pants will obviously have more than one set of numbers, depending on how many tops it matches.

- When taking off clothes, pin socks together immediately before tossing them into the laundry. This will make sorting clothes less of a chore.

- Have toenails cut by a professional manicurist. Trim fingernails under a bright light and place each hand against a dark-colored background for contrast.

- Use a talking scale.

Entranceway

- Make sure that any entrance rugs lay perfectly flat to avoid tripping.

- Entrance steps should be well illuminated and marked with iridescent tape.

Kitchen

For people coping with macular degeneration, the kitchen can be one of the most frustrating areas of the home or one of the most satisfying. If properly set up, the continued independence associated with preparing one's own food or entertaining guests can boost self-esteem and feelings of well-being.

- Use enamel paints to paint large arrows on the stove knobs to indicate On and Off positions. Buy a talking timer (see Resources). Apply raised marking tape to microwaves to indicate commonly used settings.

- Keep a hand-held, lighted magnifier on the counter to help read labels.

- Use white cups for dark liquids, such as coffee, and dark containers to store light fluids such as milk. This will make it easier to detect fluid levels.

- Use nested cups for measuring, instead of trying to read the numbers on a large measuring cup. Use different colored cups for different measurements.

- Use heavy-duty freezer bags. Label the contents and purchase date with a black marker.

- For the pantry, use plastic rather than glass containers. Label them with a black marker on white tape.

- Buy pre-sliced foods whenever possible. If meats, cheeses, or other hard objects must be sliced, use a grip device (see Resources).

- Place mixing bowls in the sink when pouring, to avoid messy cleanups.

- Keep cabinet doors and drawers fully closed at all times to avoid banging into them.

Bedroom

- Buy a clock with oversized, illuminated numbers, available from catalogs. Some even announce the time at various intervals, a feature that can be set or turned off before sleeping.

- Purchase a telephone with large, lighted numbers. Consider these phones for use throughout the house.
- Place glow-in-the-dark safety tape on stair treads, doorknobs, and flashlights.
- Have a light switch installed next to the bed, so that bedroom lights can be switched on without having to leave the bed.
- Before going to bed, always be sure that there are no obstructions between the bed and the bathroom.
- Sit when dressing or undressing to minimize the risk of falling.

Special Devices

As technology advances, specialized devices are becoming available for people with visual handicaps. Browse catalog merchants and Internet sites frequently for new products.

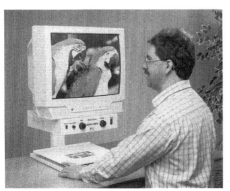

- Check with community social service agencies about obtaining a closed-circuit television (CCTV) device. These miniature video cameras allow a person to focus on bills, letters, newspapers, or magazines and enlarge them on a television screen to a comfortable magnification.
- Also, take advantage of the resources local libraries may have to make life more comfortable. Books on tape can truly help lift one's spirits. There are also magazines and newspapers available on tape.

Desktop electronic magnifiers, also known as closed-circuit televisions (cctv) offer high contrast magnification *Photo courtesy of Magnisight and the VisAbility Center.*

100

- A simple magnifying glass takes on added value when tethered to a stand, leaving both hands free. These items are available in many sizes from catalog merchants. One small caveat, however: to prevent fires, be sure not to leave magnifiers on a table that gets direct sunlight.

- While a television could hardly be called a specialized device, there are ways to make television viewing easier for people with macular degeneration. Consider a black-and-white television, which offers better contrast and may therefore be easier to see. Purchase as large a viewing screen as possible. Use a remote control device with lighted, oversized buttons.

- Catalogs offer large-format and talking devices for common items such as wristwatches, clocks, and calculators. Computers can be fitted for low vision with specialized keyboards and screen enlargers. Software programs allow enlargement of print and icons. Popular voice recognition programs such as IBM's ViaVoice or Dragon's Naturally Speaking allow the user to manipulate a computer by voice. However, they require a significant investment in time to use properly. Optical recognition programs allow the user to scan documents into a computer and enlarge them for viewing.

Household Chores

- Arrange furniture to allow obstacle-free navigation throughout the house. Make sure to tell relatives and guests the importance of not moving furniture. Keep all cabinet doors closed at all times.

- Clean windows and storm doors with a regular pattern of up-and-down, then across, to be certain that the entire surface is cleaned.

- Eliminate clutter to avoid tripping or misplacing items. Buy plastic bins and clearly label them for bills, church notices, or other purposes.

- For infirm individuals, use magnets attached to a stick to pick up metal objects or purchase a mechanical grabbing device.

- Use a steamer rather than an iron for clothing. If an iron must be used, buy one that shuts off automatically.

- Order raised-letter or large-print checks from the bank. Use pay-by-phone or Web-based payment options whenever possible.

- Keep as organized as possible. Have special locations for important items like keys, jewelry, and bills.

Recreation

- Buy large-print playing cards and board games.

- Several suppliers offer self-threading needles for household mending jobs, needlepoint, and cross-stitching.

- Instead of writing letters, use a cassette recorder and exchange tapes with friends and relatives.

- Enlarge crossword and other word puzzles on a photocopy machine.

- Finally, join a low-vision support group, often available through local hospitals or through one of the resources listed in the Resources section of this book. People who participate in these groups enjoy the support of others who face the same challenges and find wonderful tips for living life more fully.

10

Accommodations in the Workplace

Macular degeneration most often strikes after the age of 55, when people are at the peak of their careers. As a result, accommodating the workplace to valued employees with macular degeneration is often essential for a company to be able to retain the skills and experience it needs to stay competitive. In fact, many writers, artists, and businesspeople remain productive throughout their lives, long after developing macular degeneration.

The devices mentioned in this chapter, both low- and high-tech, are available through businesses listed in the Resources section of this book.

Be Informed

The Americans with Disabilities Act (ADA) of 1990 grants broad employment rights to people with disabilities. People with macular degeneration qualify under ADA guidelines, under the category of legally blind or low-vision disabilities.

Title I of the ADA makes it illegal for an employer to discriminate against otherwise qualified people with disabilities. The law also requires employers to make reasonable accommodations for such employees, unless such accommodations would pose undue financial difficulties on the employer.

A key employment trend of the past two decades has been the steady rise in home-based businesses. As these small-business people reach the age of 55, some of them will eventually be diagnosed with macular degeneration and will be faced with adapting their home offices to their disease. Whether working out of the home or in a commercial office, people with macular degeneration can organize their workplace to continue to contribute meaningfully to business, government, and nonprofit entities.

Communicate to Ease the Burden

The most essential ingredient for making a smooth transition is solid communication between the employee and management. The best way to accommodate a visually handicapped individual is for the employee and employer to communicate clearly and then to collaborate to design effective solutions. After all, most people (whether visually handicapped or not) want to be as productive as possible, and most employers want to maximize the skills and talents of all their employees.

Effective solutions often involve a staged approach that parallels vision loss. In other words, a business may not need to immediately invest in the most elaborate system available. Rather, employee and employer should discuss what accommodations are needed for the current level of visual loss, then design solutions for that level. If visual loss increases, additional solutions may be needed to accommodate the individual.

Accommodating the Workplace

Lighting

Proper lighting is absolutely essential for a person with macular degeneration to be able to perform at optimal levels at work. The two variables that must be controlled are glare and intensity. Glare should be minimized by using shades, blinds, curtains, or screens. Light intensity should be increased, particularly directly over work areas. Halogen reading lights that can be focused directly over the area being used are best for people with macular degeneration.

Organization

"Everything in its place" takes on added meaning in the workplace for a person with macular degeneration. Employees with macular degeneration should encourage coworkers to understand how important it is to label items in large letters, return items immediately to their assigned place, and to avoid clutter in general. For their part, people with macular degeneration should serve as good examples by keeping their work areas organized and free of clutter.

Navigation

Together with coworkers, employees with macular degeneration should help devise a work-flow plan that optimizes their performance. Office space should be rearranged for navigating ease. This may require relocation of the employee with macular degeneration to make common office tasks (such as photocopying) easier. After meetings, chairs should be replaced to avoid tripping.

Visual Aids

For employees with mild to moderate low vision, many large-print books, magazines, and newspapers are available to help them keep up with emerging trends in their fields. Many information sources are available through the World Wide Web. As such, they can be downloaded into a computer, picked up by a software program, and enlarged on-screen.

Similarly, clocks, calendars, calculators, and other office machines are available with large-print lettering. An employee with low vision can also use inexpensive raised-lettering machines to label items in the office.

As archaic as it sounds in today's high-tech world, a simple magnifier, especially one with a built-in light, is exceptionally helpful to a low-vision employee.

Closed-circuit television (CCTV) is a boon to people with low vision. Items like reports or magazine articles can be shown on-screen and enlarged more than twenty-five times. Contrast can also be adjusted, a helpful feature for people with macular degeneration.

Computers today are available with screen enlargement software, large-letter keyboard overlays, and voice recognition software. Optical scanners and optical recognition software are widely available and increasingly accurate. They allow a person with low vision to scan in items and enlarge them on-screen.

The Career Decision

The availability of adaptive technologies today gives people with macular degeneration unprecedented opportunities to maintain active careers. The future holds even brighter promise, as new and emerging technologies are applied to human visual pathways. In any event, thousands of employees with macular degeneration are making important contributions to their workplace every day. People with macular degeneration should be encouraged to assume active, productive careers.

11

Travel and Recreation

Coping with the effects of macular degeneration is difficult enough. It does not have to be made even more difficult by keeping oneself from enjoying the benefits of travel and recreation. Thousands of visually impaired people travel every day locally, regionally, and to distant points of the globe. Tens of thousands more enjoy recreational sports, going to the theater, or exercising to stay healthy.

Attitude is the key difference between those with macular degeneration who travel and enjoy recreational activities and those who stay home. With the abundance of resources that are available to visually handicapped people, there are few legitimate excuses for not enjoying some of life's more pleasurable pursuits.

Here are some suggestions for people with macular degeneration who wish to travel and get out more for recreational activities. They are gleaned from patients with macular degeneration who have successfully overcome some of the barriers that visually handicapped people face every day. Taking part in these activities adds significantly to one's quality of life and to one's ability to manage macular degeneration.

Travel

General Tips

- Take written directions with you so that someone can read them when offering help.

- Always carry a strong flashlight with fresh batteries.

- Keep medicines, toiletries, and other necessities with you inside a carry-on when you travel. If manageable, having an extra set of clothes in the carry-on can come in handy when luggage is misplaced. Be sure the luggage fits the carry-on restrictions of the airline.

- Use a travel agency that specializes in travel for the impaired or one that has an agent experienced in this area of travel. Several travel agencies in the United States specialize in tours for visually impaired persons. Directories of these agencies are available, both in print and on-line (see Resources). Some of these agencies mail out free newsletters describing trips and offering travel tips and safety alerts.

- Always check with final destinations to see if they offer special rates or discount coupons for impaired visitors.

- Learn to distinguish coins by their size and feel. Keep smaller-denomination bills separate from larger bills and keep them handy for tips. Fold bills differently in order to distinguish among them.

- Learn new ways to start a conversation. Like anything new, it may take some practice and a few miscues to get it "right."

- Use well-known tactics to minimize injury while walking, such as keeping your forearm slightly extended in front of you to absorb the shock of collisions, asking for help at intersections, and relying more on hearing. (See the Resources for a list of organizations that offer safety tips for the visually impaired.)

Public Transportation (Airports, Trains, and Buses)

- Plan ahead. Call or write all airline, train, or bus companies to arrange specialty handling, seating arrangements, meals, shuttle, and other services. All requests should be made at least forty-eight hours in advance. Also plan for earlier than normal check-in.
- Request pre-boarding.
- Use bright tape or a brightly colored luggage strap to better spot luggage. These are available inexpensively at travel stores or superstores.
- Use an auto-focus camera when taking pictures. Ask a friendly tourist to take a few pictures for you. Then, choose a larger-format print option when pictures are developed.

Travel Dress

- Wear a wide-brimmed hat. Studies show that a wide-brimmed hat can cut sun to the eyes by as much as 50 percent.
- Wear sunglasses that control glare (see chapter 5). Many products are available that surround the eye, providing excellent protection.
- Wear clothes with large pockets to quickly store large sunglasses or other visual aids.

Lodging

- When booking a hotel on your own, be sure to call the hotel directly, not their national 800-number. Only the hotel staff on site will be able to describe and guarantee that a room is accessible and meets the special needs of the visually impaired.

- Always keep a flashlight with fresh batteries next to the bed.

- Put reflective tape or a reflective card on the hotel room door, next to the doorknob or lock. Using a flashlight, the tape will be spotted more quickly in an emergency.

- When an unexpected visitor knocks on the door, call the front desk immediately and ask for someone to come to the room to identify the individual. Be sure to get the name of the staff person the front desk will be sending.

Recreation

Home

- Order (from specialty catalogs) board games that are created especially for the visually impaired.

- There is no need to give up activities such as crossword puzzles or other word games. Simply use a photocopy machine to enlarge them. Similarly, enlarge sheet music to continue playing musical instruments.

- Painting is a terrific hobby for sight-impaired individuals. Claude Monet continued to paint long after his vision deteriorated. Paint large. Take frequent breaks to move away from the canvas and get a better perspective on the work.

- Video games are now available for the visually impaired (see Resources).

- If walking in your neighborhood presents undue risks, or you live in a rural area, consider a low-impact exercise machine in the house such as a stair-stepper, walking machine, or elliptical trainer.

Garden

Gardening is often a lifelong pursuit that brings great pleasure to seniors. There is no need to curtail gardening activities because of macular degeneration, so long as they are planned well. One of the key difficulties with gardening is safety. The grass may be wet, rocks may be slippery, the garden path uneven, or a plant border high enough to present a tripping hazard. Here are some strategies to make your garden safe.

- Create a stone path using non-slippery surfaces, such as precast concrete. Make sure the path is even.
- Do not use borders along plantings. Instead, use a wide, thick mulch layer to delineate the path from the beginning of the plantings. In fact, the use of raised beds works best for people with macular degeneration, since they don't have to stoop as much to do their planting, weeding, and maintenance.
- Use lots of mulch between rows to minimize weeding. Keep adding mulch as the season progresses.
- Plant edibles in very straight rows. That way, anything out of those rows is most likely a weed.
- If you plant a flower garden, leave lots of space between plantings and mulch heavily. This minimizes weeds and affords easier access to the plants. Label each plant with large letters on white cardboard and place the label inside a sealable plastic bag.
- Contact the nearest agricultural extension office for tips, suggestions, and publications. Some districts have

specialists available to speak to groups of the visually impaired.

Restaurants

- When dining out, request the best-lit table in the restaurant.
- Use your flashlight to illuminate the menu. Ask the waiter or your companion to read the menu, or ask for a large-print menu.

Museums, Zoos, and Aquaria

- Arrange for special tours that allow one to touch otherwise off-limit objects. Often, a group of handicapped individuals can arrange such a trip.
- Rent the audiotaped tour of the facility, often available free to the handicapped. Many audio tours are specially produced for the visually impaired with added descriptions of the animals, paintings, or art objects.

Theaters and Movies

- Join a group that offers discussions and excursions to cultural events and places.
- Movies and videos are now available with descriptive commentary that runs parallel to the sound track and describes scenes for the visually impaired. There is even a movie reviewer who specializes in reviews for the visually impaired (see Resources).

Amusement Parks

Amusement parks throughout the country have special services for the handicapped. Call ahead to see what programs are offered for the visually impaired. Ask if they have reduced

admission fees, special grants, or discount coupons for handicapped visitors.

Gyms, Health Spas, and Bowling Alleys

- When using a gym, be sure to ask the exercise trainer for
an orientation to the equipment. Many gyms will provide
an escort at each session to accompany a visually
impaired member or visitor.
- Many modern bowling centers offer lanes with floor
markers or rails for the visually impaired.

Sports

- People with macular degeneration may not need to give
up golf, although their handicap may increase. There are
golf programs throughout the country that cater to
low-vision players. Using high-contrast golf balls can
sometimes help. Ask a golfing partner to help spot the
golf ball.
- Dancing, swimming, or bicycling on a tandem bicycle are
wonderful activities for the sight impaired.

12

A Ten-Step Prevention Program

Individuals can reduce their risk of losing vision from macular degeneration, and minimize further damage if some vision has already been lost, by practicing a ten-step prevention program based on scientific evidence. Following such a program should also help improve overall eye health as well as overall body health.

The steps mentioned here have been covered in detail in this book. However, it is useful to have the entire prevention program outlined in one place, to serve as an overview.

Remember, a good prevention program begins with an effective monitoring plan to detect changes in vision. The earlier macular degeneration is detected, the greater the number of treatment options and the greater the chances for successful treatment.

Step 1: Implement an Effective Monitoring Program
- Check each eye individually with the Amsler Grid.
- Test daily.
- Test both near and far vision.
- Document a baseline pattern.
- Understand changes and their relevance.

Step 2: Note and Report Changes in Vision

- Note changes in vision on the Amsler Grid.
- Document those changes on a fresh Amsler Grid.
- Report any changes to the doctor or medical office staff *immediately.*
- Develop a common language with your doctor to describe symptoms (i.e. blurring, blotches, blank spots, distortion).
- Create a communication plan with your doctor.
- Agree on a point of contact.
- Develop a good relationship with your doctor.
- Take an active role in your care.

Step 3: Organize an Effective Schedule of Eye Exams

- Schedule regular professional eye exams.
- Keep to the schedule of professional exams.
- If the schedule is disrupted, call the doctor and discuss what to do.
- Even if a professional eye exam is only a week or two away, call the doctor immediately if you notice any symptoms of macular degeneration.

Step 4: Assess Your Risk

- Know your family history.
- Be familiar with other risk factors.
- Take the risk self-assessment in this book.

Step 5: Optimize Nutrition

- Take control of your diet.
- Eat a balanced diet rich in vegetables and grains.
- Eat *at least* one serving a day of green leafy vegetables.
- Control the amount of dietary fats and cholesterol.
- Maintain optimal caloric intake.
- Consult with a primary care physician before making any significant dietary changes.

Step 6: Change Risky Health Habits

- Stop smoking.
- Exercise.
- Use alcohol in moderation.
- Get regular medical checkups.

Step 7: Screen Out the Sun

- Buy quality sunglasses that filter blue and UV light.
- Wear a wide-brimmed hat.
- Always use sunscreen.

Step 8: Understand and Participate in Treatment Decisions

- Understand all treatment options.
- Ask questions.
- Keep abreast of new developments.
- Be skeptical of miracle cures or exaggerated claims.

Step 9: Partner with an Experienced Retinal Specialist

- Choose an experienced retinal specialist.
- Build a strong relationship.
- Communicate any changes in vision.

Step 10: Live Well

- Value oneself and one's health.
- Quit smoking and/or excessive alcohol use.
- Eat right.
- Exercise.
- Enjoy friends and family.
- Engage spirituality.
- Cultivate a positive attitude about life.

People who implement this ten-step program will, in a short period of time, decrease their risk of losing vision from macular degeneration, improve the general health of their eyes, and feel better overall.

Appendix

Eye Diseases That Might Be Confused with Macular Degeneration

Disease	Brief Description	You have a higher risk if you:	Symptoms	Treatment	Prognosis
Macular Hole	Microscopic hole suddenly appears in center of macula	Are a woman; had a previous eye injury; had a previous macular hole; have myopia or diabetic retinopathy	Distorted vision; central black spot; blurred vision; symptoms of macular degeneration	Surgery	Excellent if damage is detected early
Macular Pucker	Thin membrane grows on retina and scar tissue forms, causing puckers	Had a detachment of the vitreous or a retinal detachment	Central vision distortion; blurred vision; double vision	Drops used to reduce swelling; surgical peeling of scar tissue	Good if not progressive; if progressive, surgery is needed to improve vision
Myopic Degeneration	Rare disorder found in severely myopic people	Have severe myopia (more than 7 or 8 diopter corrections)	Similar to macular degeneration, with visual distortion, blurring, and central gray or black spot	Similar to macular degeneration, but can sometimes be more difficult to treat	Variable
Diabetic Retinopathy	Leakage from blood vessels within the retina, as opposed to below the retina in macular degeneration; can cause scarring or complex retinal detachments	Have diabetes that is not well controlled; have had diabetes for more than 10 years; have diabetes and high blood pressure or high blood cholesterol	Blurring of vision; floaters or cobwebs in visual field; sudden and severe loss of vision	Laser used to seal leaking blood vessels; surgery may be needed to peel scars	Excellent if diabetes is controlled and early treatment is sought

Disease	Brief Description	You have a higher risk if you:	Symptoms	Treatment	Prognosis
Macular Dystrophies	Abnormalities in the cells of the retina cause symptoms similar to macular degeneration at an early age	Have a family history of the disease	Decreased vision beginning as a teenager; impaired color vision; symptoms progress slowly	No treatments currently available	Guarded
Ocular Histoplasmosis	Scars in the choroid resulting from an infection as a child by the histoplasmosis fungus	Have lived in endemic areas	Identical to macular degeneration	Use of steroids; laser, sub-retinal surgery	Somewhat better prognosis than patients with macular degeneration
Angioid Streaks	Crack-like irregularities appearing in Bruch's membrane	Had a skin disease called pseudoxanthoma elasticum; have Paget's disease or sickle-cell disease	Identical to symptoms of macular degeneration	Identical to macular degeneration	Guarded
Idiopathic Macular Degeneration	Extremely rare type of macular degeneration mostly affecting people in their 20s and 30s	Unsure of risk factors	Identical to macular degeneration	Identical macular degeneration, plus submacular surgery	Good, since patients are typically younger
Central Serous Chorio-retinopathy	A malfunction in the retinal pigment epithelium allows fluid to leak under the retina, causing a retinal detachment	Are 25-55 years old; male; type A personality	Blurred vision	Wait for spontaneous recovery; if not, laser treatments	Excellent

Resources

On-Line Resources

The following Web sites offer information about eye diseases, including treatment options and helpful advice for coping with vision loss.

All About Vision
www.allaboutvision.com
Help for individuals suffering from macular degeneration or other vision impairments. Includes a products guide.

Dr. Koop
www.drkoop.com
A site originally developed in conjunction with Dr. C. Everett Koop, the former U.S. surgeon general. Includes information on macular degeneration.

The Eye Site
www.i-care.net
Nutritional eye research summaries. Frequently asked questions, including recommended medications and nutrition.

InteliHealth
www.intelihealth.com
Includes basic information about macular degeneration, the Amsler grid, new treatments, and links to other resources.

Mayo Clinic
www.mayoclinic.com or www.mayohealth.org
User-friendly site run by one of the finest health institutions in the world. Includes information on macular degeneration, treatments, and related topics.

Medicine Net
> www.medicinenet.com
> A commercial health site with information about macular degeneration.

National Institutes of Health—Medline Plus
> www.nlm.nih.gov/medlineplus/
> User-friendly, "choose a topic by category," site. Lists resources and links to research articles. Topics include prevention, screening, diagram of the eye, treatment, and helpful organizations.

New York Online Access to Health (Ask NOAH)
> www.noah-health.org
> Sponsored by various New York organizations, including the New York library system and the New York Academy of Medicine, this site offers a potpourri of information and low-vision aids. Resources include tips on daily living and advice for caregivers. Information in English and Spanish.

USDA
> www.usda.gov
> www.healthfinder.gov
> Provides consumers with easy access to accurate on-line, health information. Links to all government nutritional-related databases.

Web MD
> www.webmd.com
> One of the most comprehensive of the commercial health sites on the Web. Includes information on macular degeneration.

Wired Seniors
> www.wiredseniors.com
> Fun and practical site that offers links to information about retinal diseases, along with other services.

Helpful Organizations

The following organizations provide helpful resources to consumers with visual impairment.

American Academy of Ophthalmology
> Public Information Program
> P.O. Box 7424
> San Francisco, CA 94120-7424
> 415-561-8555 Ext. 223
> www.eyenet.org

Provides brochures and fact sheets on eye conditions and visual impairment. Web site has a comprehensive database of information about eye diseases and conditions, including up-to-date information on nutrition, treatment, and prevention.

American Council of the Blind

1155 15th Street NW, Suite 1004
Washington, D.C. 20005
800-424-8666
202-467-5081
www.acb.org

A membership organization that advocates for the blind and visually impaired. Offers an information and referral service on all aspects of visual impairment and blindness. Web site includes many resources for the visually impaired, including medical information on macular degeneration, catalogs, books, and related links.

American Foundation for the Blind

11 Penn Plaza, Suite 300
New York, NY 10001
800-232-5463
212-502-7600
212-502-7662 TDD (for hearing impaired)
212-502-7661 (NY residents)
www.afb.org

A national clearinghouse for information about blindness and visual impairment. Offers information for the visually impaired and publishes a *Directory of Services for Blind and Visually Impaired Persons in the U.S. and Canada.* Maintains regional offices. Web site topics include aging and vision loss, education, employment, and technology. Also offers publications and links to other resources.

American Optometric Association

23 Lindbergh Boulevard
St. Louis, MO 63141
314-991-4100
www.aoanet.org

Provides brochures on low vision and other eye problems. Web site answers questions and offers consumer information, tips, and guidelines on eye exams, eye diseases, eye care, and eyewear.

Association for Macular Diseases, Inc.
210 East 64th Street
New York, NY 10021
212-605-3719
www.macula.org
A national support group that provides members with a newsletter and a phone hot line.

Canadian National Institute for the Blind
www.cnib.ca
Offers a wealth of information and tips for living with low vision, including a handbook for caregivers. Accessible in English or French.

The Center for the Partially Sighted
12301 Wilshire Boulevard, Suite 600
Los Angeles, CA 90025
310-458-3501
www.low-vision.org
Counseling center offering support groups and counseling services for people who are vision impaired. Web site offers information about warning signs and risk factors for vision loss.

Council of Citizens with Low Vision International
800-733-2258
317-254-1332
www.cclvi.org
Serves as an advocacy group for the visually impaired and provides information on low-vision technology. Publishes a newsletter.

Division of Rehabilitation Services
Independent Living Services for Older Individuals Who Are Blind
www.state.sd.us/dhs/drs/il.htm
Federally-funded program that offers free services to those age 55 and older who have severe visual impairments. Recipients do not have to be totally blind to qualify. Program requirements vary from state to state. Log on to this Web site or contact your state's division of rehabilitation services for information.

The Foundation Fighting Blindness
www.blindness.org
An organization that funds research into retinal degenerative disease worldwide. Links to many other sites and organizations. Offers access to up-to-date information about eye diseases.

Glaser-Murphy Retina Treatment Centers
> www.glasermurphyretina.com
> An informative site developed by Dr. Bert Glaser and his staff. Posts information on macular degeneration and other retinal diseases, latest research findings on prevention and treatments, and other helpful information.

Lighthouse International
> Information and Resource Service
> 111 East 59th Street
> New York, NY 10022-1202
> 800-829-0500
> 212-821-9200
> E-mail: info@lighthouse.org
> www.eyesight@eyesight.org
> Provides information about vision impairment support groups, locating vision rehabilitation services nationwide, and free publications.

The Macula Foundation
> Sponsored by the Macula Foundation, Inc. and the Association for Macular Diseases. Provides information and support for people with macular degeneration and other macular diseases.

Macular Degeneration Foundation
> P.O. Box 9752
> San Jose, CA 95157-9752
> 888-633-3937
> 408-260-1335
> E-mail: eyesight@eyesight.org
> Conducts research and educates patients on various aspects of retinal diseases. Web site includes vision care specialists, chat room, books and tapes, research on nutrition, and links to other sites.

Macular Degeneration Help Center
> 8631 West Third Street, Suite 520E
> Los Angeles, CA 90048
> 888-430-9898
> A coalition of patients, families, and leaders in the fields of vision and aging. Toll-free number has recorded information about age-related macular degeneration, 24 hours a day, 7 days a week. Web site has information about macular degeneration, including the latest news on research and experimental treatments.

National Association for the Visually Handicapped
22 West 21st Street
New York, NY 10010
212-889-3141
E-mail: staff@navh.org
or
3201 Balboa Street
San Francisco, CA 94121
415-221-3201
www.navh.org
Health agency that provides assistance to the visually impaired. Web site includes information about services available to people with low vision, plus a large-print library-by-mail service, newsletters, and kits of information.

National Eye Institute – National Institutes of Health
2020 Vision Place
Bethesda, MD 20892-3655
301-496-5248
E-mail: 2020@nei.nih.gov
www.nei.nih.gov
Provides free information to the public about eye disease prevention, treatment, and research. Web site features research results, disease information for patients, clinical studies, low vision resources, and print and audio materials.

National Federation for the Blind
1800 Johnson Street
Baltimore, MD 21230
800-638-7518
410-659-9314
E-mail: nfb@iamdigex.net
www.nfb.org
Provides referral and job services to the blind and visually impaired, as well as literature in a variety of formats. Web site offers information about services, publications, and resources available to the blind and the vision impaired.

Prevent Blindness America
500 E. Remington Road
Schaumberg, IL 60173
800-331-2020 Information hot line

847-843-2020
www.preventblindness.org
Volunteer eye health and safety organization providing public and professional education, community programs, and research aimed at preventing blindness in America. Services include a toll-free information hot line, patient services, and vision screenings. Web site has information on macular degeneration, an Amsler grid, and news about vision issues.

Visions
120 Wall Street, 16th Floor
New York, NY 10005
212-425-2255
Offers free services to anyone over age 55 with vision problems. Services include self-help study kits, counseling, professional support systems, consumer workshops, and an information center.

Catalogs, Software, Vision Aids, and Other Products

Catalogs

Blazie Engineering's Hardware Store
A Divison of Freedom Scientific
800-444-4443
www.blazie.com
Blazie and its sister companies under the Freedom Scientific umbrella offer innovative products for people with sensory and learning disabilities, including screen-reading and magnification software, Web access software, and Braille embossers and displays.

Bossert Specialties Store
3620 East Thomas Road, Suite D-124
Phoenix, AZ 85018
800-776-5885
Order M-F, 10 a.m. to 4 p.m. Mountain Time
www.bossertspecialties.com
Optical equipment sales and service. Offers trade-ins and pre-owned CCTV systems. Has handy FAQ (frequently asked questions) section and Medicare News Center. Order on-line or by telephone.

Deluxe Check Company
3660 Victoria Street, North
Shoreview, MN 55126-2906
800-328-0304 (not for ordering)
Deluxe offers personal checks for the vision impaired. Checks are larger than normal size and printed in black ink on yellow paper. Areas to be filled in are embossed for ease in locating by touch. Deluxe also offers larger check registers and deposit tickets with embossed lines. Must be ordered through a bank or other financial institution.

HumanWare
6245 King Road
Loomis, CA 95650
800-722-3393
www.humanware.com
Company that specializes in assistive technology for persons who have difficulty reading print due to blindness, low vision, or reading disabilities. Products include computer Braille and voice systems.

Independent Living Aids, Inc.
27 East Mall
Plainview, NY 11803-4404
800-537-2118
516-752-8080
www.independentliving.com
Publishes a comprehensive catalog called *CAN-DO Products* and smaller, focused catalogs called *Highlights*. Products include magnifiers, watches, clocks, timers, calculators, and writing guides. Creative cooking accessories include colored cutting boards for use with different-colored food and a six-ingredient-only cookbook. Other items offered are personal care products, computer-related items such as Braille and large-print stickers for computer keyboards, CCTVs, reading machines, and specialized computer software. Easy on-line ordering.

Independent Living Products
6227 N. 22nd Drive
Phoenix, AZ 85015-1955
800-377-8033
602-249-0455
www.ilp-online.com

Products to help the handicapped with the activities of daily living. Low-vision aids include writing aids, recreation items, magnifying tweezers, needle threaders, bent-nose pliers with adjustable magnifier, and talking calculators.

LS&S Group, Inc.

P.O. Box 673
Northbrook, IL 60065
800-468-4789
800-317-8533 TTY
www.lssgroup.com/home.html
Specializes in products for the vision and hearing impaired. Products include watches, large-print and talking dictionaries, Braille embossers, magnification products, CCTVs, talking and large-display blood pressure meters, bath and shower accessories, a variety of telephones, security devices, and universal TV remote controls. Download a catalog or call toll-free to order one.

Maxi-Aids

42 Executive Boulevard
Farmingdale, NY 11735
800-522-6294
631-752-0521
www.maxiaids.com
Publishes a comprehensive catalog featuring computer-related items, clocks, watches, calculators, electronic organizers, magnification aids, large-print playing cards, Monopoly and Scrabble, talking appliances, a large-print check register, and a host of other useful items. Easy on-line ordering.

National Association for the Visually Handicapped

22 West 21st Street
New York, NY 10010
212-889-3141
www.navh.org/shop
Offers a low-vision aids store catalog. Fax or on-line ordering.

Outa Sight Products

269 South Beverly Drive, Suite 321
Beverly Hills, CA 90212
888-876-4733
www.outa-sight.com

Variety of innovative household products for the vision impaired. Handy kitchen helpers include a "boil alert" disk, Brailled ceramics, and a "smart plug" to help in using electrical outlets.

The Rose Resnick Lighthouse Adaptations On-line Catalog
214 Van Ness Avenue
San Francisco, CA 94102
415-431-1481
415-431-4572 TTY
Fax orders to 415-863-7568
This catalog specializes in low-vision aids and offers an assortment of useful gadgets, including clocks, drawing kits, talking thermometers (ambient and fever), sewing and cooking aids, nail guides for the do-it-yourselfer, padlocks, liquid level indicators, and other useful items. Catalogs are available in Braille and large print, and on cassette and disc. No on-line ordering yet. Fax or call in orders.

Sight Connection
Community Services for the Blind and Partially Sighted
9709 Third Avenue NE #100
Seattle, WA 98115-2027
800-458-4888
Order M-F, 9 a.m. to 5 p.m. Pacific Time
206-525-5556
Catalog of clever gadgets and tools for the vision impaired. Items include talking microwave, large-print crossword puzzles, address books and check registers, tactile rulers and talking scales. Order on-line or by telephone.

The Wright Stuff
301 Alden Cove Drive
Smyrna, TN 37167
877-750-0376
www.thewright-stuff.com
Included in their catalog of items for the handicapped and arthritis sufferers are handy items for the vision impaired.

Sunglasses

Here are some of the major manufacturers of good quality, high-tech sunglasses, along with their toll-free telephone numbers and Web site addresses. Most of these companies prepare prescription sunglasses. Some specialty retail stores, such as Sunglass Hut, keep technical specifications on all sunglasses they sell. Browse several of the Web sites below to become a more knowledgeable consumer before shopping for a pair of high-quality sunglasses.

Bolle
9200 Cody
Overland Park, KS 66214
303-327-2200
www.bolle.com

Hobie
24825 Del Prado
Dana Point, CA 92629
1-888-HOBIE21
www.hobie.com

Ray-Ban Sun Optics
One Bausch & Lomb Place
Rochester, NY 14604-2701
800-343-5594
www.ray-ban.com

Revo
Luxottica SpA
Loc. Valcozzena
32021 Agordo (Belluno) - Italy
Tel. + 39.0437.6441
www.luxottica.it/english/lines/revo.htm
or
Www.lenscrafters.com

Oakley
　　1 Icon
　　Foothill Ranch, CA 92610
　　800-403-7449
　　www.oakley.com

Vuarnet Optical
　　5440 McConnell Avenue
　　Los Angeles, California 90066
　　800-348-0388
　　www.vuarnet.com

Maui Jim
　　One Aloha Lane
　　Peoria, IL 61615
　　1-888-628-4546
　　www.mauijim.com

SunTiger
　　23945 Calabasas Road, Suite 201
　　Calabasas, CA 91302
　　818-225-7765
　　www.suntigers.com

NYX Golf
　　15936 Midway Road
　　Addison, TX 75001
　　800-505-4699
　　www.nyxgolf.com

Recreation

Reading Materials

American Printing House for the Blind, Inc.
　　1839 Frankfort Avenue
　　P.O. Box 6085
　　Louisville, KY 40206-0085
　　800-223-1839
　　www.aph.org

Offers a wide variety of Braille, large-type, recorded, computer disk, and tactile publications, as well as a wide assortment of educational and daily living products. Also offers synthetic speech and enlarged-screen computer software for the visually impaired. Order either by telephone or on their Web site.

Books on Tape, Inc.
P.O. Box 7900
Newport Beach, CA 92658-7900
800-626-3333
www.booksontape.com
Provides a 30-day rental or purchase program of full-length books, from classics to best-sellers.

Choice Magazine Listening
85 Channel Drive
Port Washington, NY 11050-2216
516-883-8280
E-mail: choicemag@aol.com
www.choicemagazinelistening.org
Subscribers receive, free and bimonthly, eight hours of unabridged magazine articles, fiction, and poetry read by professional voices and recorded on four-track cassette tapes. The special-speed cassette players can be ordered free from the Library of Congress talking book program.

Doubleday Large-Print Home Library
Membership Services Center
6550 East 30th Street
P.O. Box 6325
Indianapolis, IN 46206
317-541-8920
www.doubledaylargeprint.com/
Provides hardcover editions of best-sellers in large print.

Library of Congress: National Library Service for the Blind and Physically Handicapped
1219 Taylor Street NW
Washington, D.C. 20542
800-424-8567
202-707-5100
202-707-0744 TDD
E-mail: nls@loc.gov

www.lcweb.loc.gov/nls
Administers a national library service that provides Braille and recorded books and magazines on free loan to anyone who cannot read standard print because of visual or physical disabilities. Loans are made through regional libraries only. Contact the service to locate the regional library serving your area.

National Association for the Visually Handicapped
22 West 21st Street
New York, NY 10010
212-889-3141
E-mail: staff@navh.org
www.navh.org
Offers a large-print loaning library by mail and a quarterly newsletter.

New York Times/Large-Print Weekly
229 West 43rd Street
New York, NY 10036
800-631-2580 Phone orders
Offers weekly subscriptions to the *New York Times* in large print.

Reader's Digest Large-Print Edition
P.O. Box 3010
Harlan, IA 51593-0101
800-807-2780
Offers subscription to large-print monthly edition of *Reader's Digest* magazine. Each issue includes all the favorite sections, illustrated in bold and in color on non-glare paper.

Reader's Digest Large-Print Reader
P.O. Box 262
Mount Morris, IL 61054
800-877-5293
Offers yearly, 6-volume subscriptions of choice reading from *Reader's Digest Select* editions. Each volume contains two stories selected from popular mysteries, comedies, adventure tales, etc. All in easy-to-read large type on non-glare paper.

Thorndike Press
P.O. Box 159
Thorndike, ME 04986-0159
800-223-1244 Phone orders and customer service
800-558-4676 Fax orders

E-mail orders: galeord@galegroup.com
www.mlr.com/thorndike
Offers a large selection of large-print books. Send mail orders to the
above address, or call the 800 number.

Travel

Access-Able Travel Source
Provides detailed information for mature and disabled travelers, including
specialized travel agencies and tours, as well as packing and travel tips.
Has links to many other related Web sites. Also posts travel stories.

Accessible Tours
A Division of Directions Unlimited
123 Green Lane
Bedford Hills, NY 10507
800-533-5343
914-241-1700
Specializes in both domestic and international travel tours for the
handicapped.

The Campanian Society
Box 167
Oxford, OH 45056
513-524-4846
www.campanian.org
Offers tours that do not rely on sight but on the other four senses.
Previous tours have included the monuments of Washington, D.C., the
sandwich glass factories of Cape Cod, and the beaches of Key West.

Directory of Travel Agencies for the Disabled
Twin Peaks Press
Box 129
Vancouver, WA 98666-0129
800-637-2256 To order
360-694-2462 For information
Handbook of travel resources written by Helen Hecker, R.N., which can
be ordered through Twin Peaks Press. Twin Peaks also offers a catalog of
helpful books in their "Disability Bookshop."

The Guided Tour, Inc.
7900 Old York Road
Suite 114-B
Elkins Park, PA 19027-2339
800-783-5841
215-782-1370
www.guidedtour.com
Offers professionally supervised travel and vacation programs for persons with developmental and physical challenges. For most persons with visual handicaps, they have a 1:1 staff-to-traveler ratio.

Miscellaneous

Blind Sports and Recreation Resources, accessed through the Mississippi State University Research and Training Center on Blindness and Low Vision
www.blind.msstate.edu
Part of a comprehensive database of on-line resources that provide information about blindness and low vision as part of Mississippi State's Information and Resource Referral Project. This link lists recreational resources for the vision impaired from baseball and golf to skiing and scuba diving.

Blindspots
www.vashti.net/blind/
Rates movies for the blind and visually impaired. The reviewer rates movies on a scale from 1 to 10, from being impossible to follow even with a sighted assistant, to a movie that a visually impaired person could follow without any assistance. Usually, a rating of 6 or higher will be workable with a sighted assistant. As noted on the Web site, the reviewer makes no judgments about profanity, violence, or sexuality, only the ease or difficulty that visually impaired people will experience while following the story.

Guitar by Ear
704 Habersham Rd
Valdosta, GA 31602
800-484-1839
229-249-0628
Sells learning programs to learn guitar or piano by ear.

MindsEye2

Route 1, Box 404-A
Bland, VA 24315
www.mindweye2.com
Catalog of computer games for the vision impaired. Many are for children, but many are for families and adults.

National Beep Baseball Association

c/o Jeanette Bigger, Secretary
2231 West 1st Street
Topeka, KS 66606
785-234-2156
www.nbba.org.
Start a Beep Baseball team or check out the history of the game. Beep Baseball enables the blind and vision impaired to enjoy playing baseball.

Glossary

A

    Alternative Medicine: Healing practices other than those of mainstream medicine.

    Amblyopia: An imbalance between a person's eyes during early childhood that leads to permanent loss of vision.

    Americans with Disabilities Act (ADA): A federal law that grants certain rights to disabled individuals.

    Amsler Grid: A grid with a dot in the center, used to test for symptoms that may signify macular degeneration.

    Angiography: The process of obtaining images of blood vessels within and under the retina that retinal surgeons use to determine how best to stop them from leaking.

    Angioid Streaks: Crack-like irregularities that appear in Bruch's membrane.

    Antioxidant: An agent that reduces the damage due to by-products of the normal chemical reactions with oxygen in the body.

    Apheresis: A procedure used to remove harmful substances from the blood.

    Arteriosclerosis: Thickening of the walls of the arteries.

    Artery: Blood vessel that carries oxygenated blood to the tissues of the body.

    Atherosclerosis: The accumulation of fatty deposits on the walls of large blood vessels.

B

    Blank Spots: A commonly reported symptom of macular degeneration in which patients report that areas of their view disappear.

Blotches: A commonly reported symptom of macular degeneration in which patients report that gray or black stains appear in their view.

Blue Light: A portion of the light spectrum that is suspected of being harmful to the retina.

Blurring: A commonly reported symptom of macular degeneration in which patients report that lines or edges of objects lose their sharpness.

Braille: A system of raised letters. People who are legally blind read by touching the letters with their fingers.

Bruch's Membrane: A thin, compact layer of fibers located between the retina and the underlying flat carpet of blood vessels that supplies the retina with nourishment.

C

Cataract: A clouding of the lens that causes decreased vision.

CCTV (Closed-circuit television): A technology that uses a video camera to place objects on a screen at increased magnification.

Central Atrophy: A thinning of the retina that occurs as part of macular degeneration.

Central Serous Retinopathy: A malfunction of the retinal pigment epithelium that allows fluid to leak under the retina, causing a limited retinal detachment.

Cholesterol: A waxy substance that can accumulate on the walls of arteries and cause health problems. The body produces all the cholesterol it needs without adding any to the diet.

Choroid: Nnetwork of blood vessels under the retina.

Classic Choroidal Neovascularization: A type of wet macular degeneration characterized by rapid leaking of fluids under the retina and rapidly appearing visual problems.

Compliance: Carefully following the recommendations of health-care providers.

Conjunctiva: A mucus membrane that lines the inside of the eyelids and extends over the front of the white part of the eye.

Consultation: The most extensive type of medical exam.

Cornea: The transparent outermost part of the eye that helps focus the image.

Counseling: Discussions with a health-care professional regarding assistance with life situations, behavior, relationships, and feelings.

D

Depression: Feelings of helplessness, hopelessness, despair, and possible thoughts of suicide.

Diabetes: An abnormality of insulin production that results in elevated blood sugar. The elevated blood sugar can cause damage to many organs of the body, including the retina.

Diabetic Retinopathy: Leaking of blood vessels within the retina, commonly found in diabetics, that can lead to retinal swelling, scarring, and retinal detachment. All of these abnormalities can be prevented in most cases if treatment is instituted early, before symptoms occur.

Diagnose: To determine the cause of an illness or medical condition.

Dietician: Health-care worker trained to consult patients on daily food intake and diet.

Disability: An impairment that affects one's ability to perform certain daily functions.

Distortions: A commonly reported symptom of macular degeneration in which patients report that lines in their view appear wavy.

Dominant Eye: The eye that is preferred.

Double Vision (Diplopia): Vision in which a single object appears double.

Drusen: Small yellow mounds of debris that accumulate within Bruch's membrane and are often an early sign of age-related macular degeneration.

Dry Macular Degeneration: The wasting away of retinal cells most likely due to lack of nourishment and buildup of waste materials.

E

Enzyme: A special protein that acts as a promoter during chemical reactions in the body.

Experimental: Not yet proven or available for general use.

Exudate: A clear fluid.

F

Feeder Vessel Treatment: Stopping retinal bleeding by closing the blood vessels that supply the leaking blood vessels.

Glossary

Fibrosis: The process the body uses to create scar tissue.

Flashes of Light: One of the most common indications of retinal problems. However, flashes can occur without retinal problems.

Fovea: The center part of the macula that provides the sharpest vision.

Free Radicals: Toxic substances produced by all cells.

G

Gene Therapy: A method using genes (sequences of DNA) to treat disease.

Glaser Monitoring Program: A basic series of self-tests to monitor for the development or progression of macular degeneration.

Glaser Ten-step Program: A medically based program to help detect and minimize progression and damage from macular degeneration.

Glaucoma: Disorder of the eye characterized by an increase of pressure within the eyeball.

Green Leafy Vegetables: Vegetables such as spinach, kale, and swiss chard. Thought to be beneficial to the healthy functioning of the body, especially the eyes.

H

HDL (high density lipoproteins): The "good" form of cholesterol that removes LDLs from the body.

High Blood Pressure: An elevation of the pressure of blood in the arteries produced by the pumping action of the heart.

High-speed Angiography: Using a computer to obtain high-speed images in order to better detect and delineate the pattern of leaking blood vessels under the retina.

I

Idiopathic: A disease of unknown origin or without apparent cause.

Idiopathic Macular Degeneration: An extremely rare form of macular degeneration that affects people in their twenties and thirties.

Infection: Inflammation in body tissue caused by microorganisms.

Inflammation: A localized response to tissue injury characterized by swelling, redness, heat, tenderness, and loss of function.

Internship: Name given to the first year of training for surgeons just out of medical school.

Intravitreal Bubble: A gas bubble sometimes introduced into the eye to displace or stop retinal bleeding. This technique is also commonly used in the repair of retinal detachments.

Iris: The tissue in front of the lens that opens and closes to control the amount of light entering the eye. The iris is the structure that gives color to the eye.

J

K

L

Lens: The clear structure near the front of the eye that focuses images onto the retina. It has the same shape and function as the lens within a camera.

LDL (low density lipoproteins): The "bad" form of cholesterol that becomes incorporated into blood vessel walls.

Lutein: A vitamin that might reduce the risk of macular degeneration, but which has not yet been proven to do so.

M

Macula: The center of the retina. Used for direct focusing.

Macular Degeneration: An abnormality of the blood supply to the light-sensitive portion of the retina that is primarily a result of aging.

Macular Dystrophies: Abnormalities in cells of the retina that can cause symptoms of macular degeneration at an early age.

Macular Hole: A microscopic hole that can appear in the macula.

Macular Pucker: A thin membrane growing on the retina that contacts and distorts the retina, resulting in blurred and distorted vision.

Macular Translocation: A surgical procedure that relocates the macula away from leaking blood vessels.

Meditation: To engage in extended thought or contemplation as a method of reducing stress.

Metabolism: The processing of substances in the body such as food into energy or structural components.

Microscope: An instrument that provides magnified images of very tiny objects.

Microsurgery: Surgery on fine structures using magnified glasses or a microscope.

Minor Surgery: Surgery requiring any type of anesthesia, performed as an outpatient procedure or in a doctor's office, and resulting in a short recovery time.

Monounsaturated Fat: A class of oils (including olive oil and canola oil) that is better for the body than saturated or polyunsaturated fats.

Myopic Degeneration: An abnormality similar to macular degeneration that can occur in severely myopic people.

N

Nerves: Fibers containing nerve cells that convey impulses from the central nervous system to other parts of the body.

Neurologic: Referring to the nervous system.

O

Occult Choroidal Neovascularization: A type of wet macular degeneration characterized by slower leakage of fluids under the retina.

Ocular Histoplasmosis: Scars in the choroid resulting from infection by a fungus.

Operation: A procedure performed by a surgeon to remove or repair part of the body.

Ophthalmologist: Physician who specializes in the diagnosis, medical treatment, and surgical treatment of eye diseases.

Optometrist: A licensed eye caregiver who specializes in eye exams, prescribing lenses, and certain medical treatments.

Oxidation: A process in which certain by-products of oxygen use react with nearby molecules. It is thought to cause damage to tissues.

P

Photodynamic Treatment: The use of laser beams to activate special dyes in order to stop retinal bleeding.

Photokeratitis: A painful but temporary condition of the eye caused by intense light sources, such as an arc welder.

Pigment Epithelial Detachment: A split occurring in Bruch's membrane fills with fluid and causes a dome-shaped detachment of the pigment epithelium underlying the retina, leading to visual distortion or other symptoms. Pigment epithelial detachments are often associated with macular degeneration.

Pigment Epithelium Rip: A severe condition caused by a tear in the pigment epithelium, leading to sudden loss of vision. Pigment epithelial rips are often associated with macular degeneration but can also result from direct trauma to the eye.

Polypoidal Choroidal Neovascularization: Small swellings within the walls of blood vessels under the retina burst and cause damage to the retina.

Polyunsaturated Fats: Help rid the body of cholesterol, but should still be limited in one's diet.

Prognosis: The likely outcome of a disease, often given in terms of the expected outcome over a certain number of years.

Pterygium: A scarring condition of the cornea, caused by exposure to intense sunlight.

Q

R

Receptors: Sites in the brain that allow the attachment of certain drugs, making them active and able to produce the desired results.

Red Blood Cells: The cells in the blood that carry oxygen.

Remodeling: The process by which the blank spots noted by patients using the Amsler grid change positions.

Retina: The part of the eye that contains the rods and the cones. It receives the image from the lens and conveys visual information to the brain via the optic nerve. The retina functions much like the film in a camera or the chip in a video camera.

Retinal Fibrosis: Scarring in the retina.

Retinal Pigment Epithelium (RPE): a single layer of cells between the retina and the underlying blood vessels.

Retinal Surgeon: An ophthalmologist specializing in diseases of the retina.

Risk Factors: Behaviors that increase a person's risk of getting a disease.

S

Saturated Fats: Fats found in red meats and certain plants, like the coconut and palm. High levels of these fats are known to be harmful to the body and should be limited.

Second Opinion: An extensive exam designed to get input and an opinion from a second physician.

Sedation: Medication given to reduce awareness.

Side Effect: An unintended consequence of a treatment.

Sign: Observable evidence of disease.

Stem Cell: A type of primitive cell that can transform into and generate other cells.

Subretinal Hemorrhage: A condition caused by pooling of blood under the retina.

Support Group: A group of people who meet regularly to support or sustain each other by discussing common problems.

T

Tear Film: a layer of fluid which bathes and lubricates the cornea.

Tissue: Body components made of living cells.

Transfusion: The procedure of transferring blood or blood products from one person to another.

Transpupillary Thermotherapy (TTT): The use of infrared light to stop retinal bleeding.

U

Ultraviolet (UV) Light: The non-visible portion of the light spectrum with a wavelength shorter than violet light.

V

Vitamin C: A well-known antioxidant.

Vitamin E: A vitamin whose role is not clear in terms of preventive effects on the eye.

Vitreous: The clear, jelly-like fluid in the central portion of the eye.

Vitreous Hemorrhage: Hemorrhage within the vitreous of the eye.

W

Wet macular degeneration: The abnormal increase in and leaking from blood vessels under the retina, leading to disturbances of the central field of vision.

World Wide Web: A computer-accessed information system with extensive information available about most subjects.

X
Y
Z

Zeaxanthin: A vitamin that may help prevent macular degeneration, but which has not yet been proven to do so.

Zinc: An antioxidant that neutralizes free radicals and is important to the proper functioning of the body. Its role in macular degeneration is unknown.

Index

theaters, 113
travel dress, 110
zoos, 113
travel tips, 109, 110
treatment options, 79–94
TTT (transpupillary thermotherapy), 83, 84

U

ultraviolet (UV) light, 31, 32, 56, 57
U.S. Department of Agriculture, 50
U.S. Recommended Dietary Allowance (USRDA), 55
UV light protection, 57, 58
UV (ultraviolet light), 31, 32, 56, 57

V

vegetables, 45, 46
vision
blurring, 6
central, 10, 11
changes in, 4, 10, 80
distorted, 6
loss, 1
visual acuity, 21, 22
visual field testing, 22, 23

visual rehabilitation services, 67
Visudyne, 80–83
vitamins, 31, 46, 55
vitreous, 2, 25, 36
cavity, 88, 89
exam, 25
gel, 89
hemorrhaging, 9, 88–90

W

wet macular degeneration, 1
defined, 5, 6
signs, 26
symptom, 11, 12
treatment options, 80–94
types, 6–8
workplace
accommodations, 103–107
discrimination, 103
lighting, 105
navigating the office, 105
organizing the office, 105
visual aids, 106

Z

zeaxanthin, 46
zinc, 54, 55
zoos, 113

About the Authors

Bert Glaser, M.D., is an internationally respected retinal surgeon, having pioneered some of today's cutting-edge laser treatments for macular degeneration, surgical repair of macular holes, and techniques to diagnose and treat many other diseases of the retina. Dr. Glaser is a professor and director of retina at George Washington University Medical Center; he is a former professor of ophthalmology and director of vitreoretinal research at the Johns Hopkins Wilmer Eye Institute. Dr. Glaser is currently chairman and director of the Glaser Murphy Retina Treatment Centers of Baltimore, Maryland and Washington, D.C. Dr. Glaser can be contacted at www.glasermurphyretina.com.

Lester A. Picker, Ed.D., is former editor in chief of The Johns Hopkins Medical Institutions *Women's Health* line of information products and has more than 500 published credits in nationally circulated magazines and other publications. Picker is a member of the American Society of Journalists and Authors. He can be contacted at lpicker@home.com.